Everything You Always Wanted to
Ask Your Gynecologist

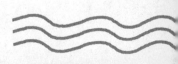

Everything You Always Wanted to
Ask Your Gynecologist

Answers to Over 200 Questions
Commonly Asked by Women

R. Scott Thornton, M.D.
and Kathleen Schramm, M.D.

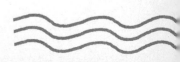

Houghton Mifflin Company
Boston • New York • 1998

For information about permission to reproduce selections
from this book, write to Permissions,
Houghton Mifflin Company, 215 Park Avenue South,
New York, New York 10003.

Library of Congress Cataloging-in-Publication Data
Thornton, R. Scott.
Everything you always wanted to ask your gynecologist :
answers to over 200 questions commonly asked by women /
R. Scott Thornton and Kathleen Schramm.
p.   cm.
Includes index.
ISBN 0-395-89262-7
1. Gynecology — Miscellanea. 2. Gynecology — Popular
works. 3. Women — Health and hygiene — Miscellanea.
4. Self-care, Health — Miscellanea. I. Schramm, Kathleen.
II. Title.
RG121.T487   1998
618.1 — dc21   98-17932 CIP

Printed in the United States of America

Book design by Joyce C. Weston
Illustrations by J/B Woolsey Associates
Cover design by Susan McClellan

QUM 10 9 8 7 6 5 4 3 2 1

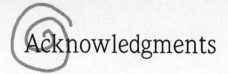Acknowledgments

We must start by thanking the many teachers who taught us writing. Teachers rarely have the opportunity to see the fruits of their labor. Without their sincere efforts, we would not have developed the ability or confidence necessary to write this book. After they have finished banging their heads against the wall at the end of the day, they need to know that they have made a difference.

Thanks also to Michelle Valentine for her initial perusal and impressions of the book. Her confidence in our work spurred us on.

Our gratitude extends to the many people at Houghton Mifflin who worked on the book. We warmly thank Rux Martin, our editor, who diligently translated medical jargon into understandable words. We would also like to thank the manuscript editor, Susanna Brougham, and the illustrator, Regina Santoro.

We are indebted to our parents for their love and support throughout this project. Thanks to our daughter, Christine, for her patience and to our son, Michael, who had to give up his computer games so Dad and Mom could write.

We especially want to thank our patients. Without your questions, there would be no book.

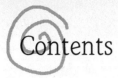

Contents

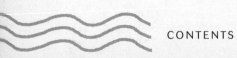

CONTENTS

treated? • Why does my doctor's treatment for dysplasia differ from the treatment received by someone I know with the same condition? • Will dysplasia come back again after treatment? • If dysplasia can recur, why isn't hysterectomy always the treatment of choice? • What's the difference between cervical dysplasia and cervical cancer? • How will I know if I have cervical cancer? • How is cervical cancer treated? • What are my chances of surviving cervical cancer?

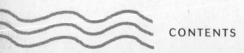

CONTENTS

When You Need Surgery (*cont.*)

as an outpatient? • How much pain will I have after laparoscopic surgery? • Can hysteroscopy be done in the office? • How much pain and bleeding will I have after hysteroscopy?

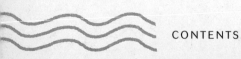

CONTENTS

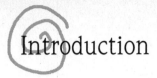Introduction

You have a question to ask a gynecologist. Maybe it's about premenstrual syndrome, or menopause, or that annoying pain that appears below your bellybutton. It isn't an emergency. Being considerate, you don't bother the doctor with a phone call. It only seems fair that you make an appointment to discuss this properly.

You nearly hit a car trying to decipher the multitude of signs outside the office building. There must be 200 names on the directory at the entrance, but eventually you find the correct office. Terrific, you're right on time.

You spend another 20 minutes completing the questionnaire handed to you by the receptionist. Who dreams up these information sheets, anyway? Even Uncle Sam doesn't get this personal. Is it really necessary to know my religion?

Finally, the nurse calls you back to an examining room. Apparently, the staff forgot to pay the heating bill. The temperature is more conducive to chilling a chardonnay than examining a naked woman. The nurse asks you to empty your bladder. She instructs you to totally disrobe. (Is it too late to back out now?) You put on a disposable gown made of tissue paper. You've been instructed to leave it open in the front. Well, you didn't really expect to maintain modesty, did you?

After an eternity, the doctor finally arrives. "Hello, I'm Dr. Stewart. What brings Eileen in today?" Now is your chance. You ask your question, and the doctor magically transforms into one of the following:

 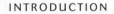

1. *The Great Evader:* He or she starts to give a reasonable reply, only to deftly switch in midresponse to a topic of no significance — one that is easier to discuss, such as the weather.
2. *The Humorist:* He or she makes light of the situation. This relieves some of the tension that naturally occurs in a sensitive discussion, but still doesn't answer your question.
3. *The Great Escape Artist:* This doctor defers the question until the end of the examination and then mumbles a perfunctory response while backing out of the door, wishing you a pleasant day.
4. *The Well-Intentioned but Desperately Short-of-Time Physician:* We hope most doctors fall into this category. They are well informed on a variety of topics pertinent to their specialty, but because of a large volume of patients, their schedule allows only 10 to 15 minutes per patient. They will do their best to give you informative answers, but often lack time to adequately address the issue.

As physicians, we empathize with both the patient and her doctor in this predicament. Periodically, we present seminars within our community. A worthy overview of almost any topic generally consumes one hour. Your doctor can't possibly spend that much time with a patient in the office on a regular basis and survive in today's medical climate — it is uncommon to schedule more than 20 minutes per patient. Brochures or videos can help educate patients, but they often don't provide enough information, and they tend to be impersonal.

We also realize that many women have questions that they never ask. Anxiety (let's be honest — going to the gynecologist is not the easiest task in the world) may cause anyone to forget to ask important questions. Some topics just seem too embarrassing to bring up. Many women deem their questions too "stupid" to ask.

With this in mind, *Everything You Always Wanted to Ask Your Gynecologist* was conceived. It is dedicated to all of the women who have walked into a gynecologist's office with a question and left with an unsatisfactory answer (or left without asking the question). We'll examine the most commonly asked questions and try to give valuable insight and advice. However, never forget that your best resource is still your personal gynecologist.

Regardless of your problem, keep in mind the following pointers when you consult a gynecologist:

1. *Don't make assumptions!* When you develop a symptom, such as unusual bleeding, pelvic pain, or vaginal discharge, don't assume that a disaster is brewing. Your symptom may not indicate a problem. Keep in mind that most gynecologic disorders are not life threatening and can be remedied. On the other hand, don't assume that your symptom is normal. Most delays in treatment occur because patients fail to seek appropriate attention.

2. *Avoid self-treatment.* It's often said, "He who treats himself has a fool for a patient." Always see a professional for evaluation and treatment. The people you hear plugging various cures over television and radio aren't paid to solve your problem. They're paid to sell a product. Using over-the-counter products without the advice of a medical professional is playing Russian roulette with your health. Likewise, this book is not intended to replace your gynecologist. It should supplement the information he or she provides and give you a basis for meaningful discussion.

3. *Educate yourself.* Educate yourself, but choose your resources carefully. We have tried to provide unbiased information in this book. Books, pamphlets, and audiovisual resources produced by the American College of Obstetrics and Gynecology or other reputable medical institutions are reliable sources of information. Your doctor may have these or other resources available in the office. Be leery of information transmitted through television news shows and magazines, which is often oversimplified or distorted.

4. *Don't be afraid to ask "dumb" questions.* Odds are pretty good that your doctor has heard the same question from many other women. Make a note of your questions when you think of them. When you get to the office, there is a good chance that you'll forget a question if it is not written down.

5. *Communicate clearly with your doctor's office.* When you call the office, state whether your problem is urgent. Your doctor will find time to see you promptly if the problem is really an emergency. But don't cry wolf. If you portray everything as an emergency, your doctor may

eventually learn to ignore your complaints. If you anticipate a lengthy visit because you have a complex problem or an extensive medical history, inform the receptionist and ask for more time. If the receptionist cannot accommodate you, ask to speak with the physician or find a new doctor.

6. *Don't compare yourself to other people.* Doctors cringe when they hear "My aunt Tilly had this same thing and her doctor said . . ." Every patient and problem presents a unique set of circumstances. Recommendations applicable to one patient may not be appropriate for another. We have also seen patients ignore recommendations because their mother (or uncle, or neighbor . . . the list goes on) didn't "think it was a good idea." If you feel uncomfortable with your doctor's recommendation, ask more questions or seek a second opinion. Don't be influenced by people — no matter how much they love you — who do not have medical credentials.

7. *Trust your doctor, but don't blindly follow the advice.* When your doctor recommends a specific treatment, he or she should explain the rationale behind it. If further clarification is necessary, ask more questions. If you still feel uncomfortable, seek a second opinion. But avoid the tendency to run around obtaining multiple "second opinions." If your doctor meets the following criteria, you are probably in good hands. He or she should

- have a good reputation among other health care professionals.
- offer rational, concise explanations for his or her recommendations.
- provide you with alternatives and options when they exist.
- have extensive experience in dealing with the disorder in question.

Without further delay, let's embark on our exploration of the world of gynecology.

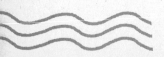

1 The Big Picture: When to See a Gynecologist

Why should I go to a gynecologist?

Having someone examine you while you are nearly naked is at best embarrassing and at worst mortifying. Why should you subject yourself to it? Well, the first and foremost reason is for cancer screening. It's amazing how many people don't even want to talk about cancer, never mind be screened for it. They have "ostrich syndrome": They believe that if they bury their heads in the sand and don't look for it, then it won't happen.

If you are destined to develop cancer, it will occur whether or not you're screened. Screening, however, helps the doctor discover it early, increasing the chances of successful treatment. A glance at the history of cervical cancer treatment clearly shows the importance of early detection. The incidence of cervical cancer in the 1950s was 30 to 35 cases per 100,000 per year in women over the age of 20. With the advent of the Pap smear (a test that detects this cancer), the incidence of cancer dropped to only 10 cases per 100,000 women — and this despite an epidemic rise in the sexual transmission of viruses that predispose women to cervical cancer. Although the media seem to be fond of locating women who develop cervical cancer in spite of screening, such problems are rare. Without a doubt, the institution of regular screening with Pap smears has been successful. At your visit you will also be screened for breast, colon, vaginal, vulvar, and ovarian cancer. We'll delve into the specifics of these conditions later.

Family planning is another important reason for consulting a gynecologist. A large number of pregnancies are accidental. Reasons given by younger women include these:

- "I didn't think I could get pregnant the first time."
- "We did it only once."
- "He said he loved me." (The "he" in question has long since left.)
- "I don't know how this happened." (This is our personal favorite.)

Unintended pregnancies also occur in the later reproductive years. Older women can be taken by surprise just like younger women:

- "But I was told I couldn't get pregnant at my age."
- "Well, we were meaning to get around to doing something more permanent about contraception."
- "I didn't think women could get pregnant this late in life."

Your best chance of having the right size family, at the right time in your life, is to practice family planning. Your gynecologist is the best person to help you in this endeavor. There are a wide variety of contraceptive options and other techniques to help you plan for the best time to have your baby.

Finally, regular appointments with your gynecologist can provide you with a greater understanding of your body and health. Throughout your life, you will face a wide range of normal and possibly abnormal developments. During your reproductive years, you may confront premenstrual syndrome, menstrual irregularities, fibroids, endometriosis, infertility, and concerns related to pregnancy. In the postreproductive years, you will go through menopause. You may also have concerns regarding bladder dysfunction or other problems related to changes in the pelvic area as you get older. As the years advance, the risk of developing cancer increases. Visiting your gynecologist on a regular basis ensures that these issues can be addressed promptly.

How should I choose a gynecologist?

Locating a competent and caring gynecologist can be a challenge. Many women find a doctor based on the recommendation of a friend or neighbor. However, such recommendations can be misleading. Doctor "X" may be very congenial, but incompetent. A general practitioner whom you trust is more qualified to suggest someone to you. If your

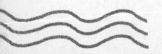

doctor is a man, ask whom his wife visits for her exams. If your general practitioner is a woman, ask her whom she sees.

If you are new to the area, first determine which of the nearby hospitals has the best reputation. Then call the hospital and ask to speak with the nurse in charge of the labor and delivery suite. He or she works with the physicians on a daily basis and should be able to make a reasonable assessment of the doctors' capabilities and "bedside manner." Also contact the nurse in charge of the operating room for an assessment of their surgical skills. Communicating with these people is more valuable than contacting the hospital's referral service. The referral service can provide you with the names of gynecologists in your vicinity but cannot comment on their level of competence.

Should you try to locate a female gynecologist? You may assume that a female gynecologist will be more empathetic in treating your problems. That is not necessarily true. Most men who choose gynecology as a profession are very personable and enjoy treating women. Often older women seek a male gynecologist, presuming that he will be more competent than a female simply because few women of their generation became physicians. Try to choose a doctor on the basis of ability and disposition, not gender. If you are particularly anxious about visiting a gynecologist and feel that you will be more comfortable seeing a woman doctor, then try to find one. Otherwise, concentrate on locating the best physician, regardless of sex.

I'm too anxious and embarrassed to see a gynecologist. What can I do?

You are not alone. Many women never, or rarely, visit a gynecologist for this very reason. The embarrassment of having a gynecologist examine you can be overwhelming. The fact that he or she examines thousands of women every year doesn't provide much consolation. You may also fear that the doctor will discover a serious problem.

Understanding the purpose of your visit may help you overcome your reservations. It will be especially important for you to choose a gynecologist who can make you feel comfortable.

To help overcome your anxiety, consider accompanying a friend on her visit to a gynecologist. The gynecologist's office will not seem as ominous if you know you are not there for an examination. Then consider making an appointment just to talk. Conversing with the doctor while you are fully clothed eases some of the tension and enables you to feel more at ease. The doctor can take your history and explain the procedures involved in an examination.

If you feel comfortable with the doctor, schedule an examination. For emotional support, consider bringing a friend who can either stay in the waiting room or come in with you during the exam. A nurse from the office can also serve in this capacity (many doctors routinely have a nurse in the room during exams; if not, you may request one).

Why do I have such a hard time getting an appointment?

You finally get through to the doctor's office after hearing busy signals all day. Well, at least you're close to getting an appointment, right? *Not!* The receptionist gives you an appointment just this side of eternity. Why? Most good physicians have a backlog of routine appointments. They have developed a large base of patients, and other doctors refer additional patients to them as well. Therefore the appointment schedule may extend well into the future. It is critically important to communicate clearly to the receptionist if your problem is urgent. She or he usually will add you to the next office session. For a true emergency, be prepared to visit the emergency room. If you think your problem demands prompt attention and the receptionist seems to be putting you off, leave your name and phone number. Ask for the physician to call you back at the earliest convenience. You can then discuss the situation. If it is necessary, the doctor will find a way to see you. If you prefer a specific date or time for a routine appointment, call the office well in advance. Usually your request can be honored.

When is the best time to schedule an appointment?

It depends on what type of visit is necessary. When an extensive discussion of a topic is required, inform the receptionist while scheduling your appointment. Extra time can be allotted. Inquire as to the best point in the schedule for a lengthy discussion. This may be the last appointment of the day. You will possibly have to wait longer (if the doctor is behind schedule), but at least you will have more time to talk. This

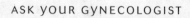

ASK YOUR GYNECOLOGIST

applies only if the doctor does not have surgery or an important meeting scheduled after hours, so check with the staff. When you come, bring a written list of your concerns and questions. Time is valuable, so stay on the subject of your health care and avoid small talk.

Ideally, you should not schedule an appointment on a day that the doctor covers deliveries. If a woman in labor needs attention, the doctor will be eager to finish the office session. You also run the risk that the doctor will leave for a delivery in the middle of office hours, which really fouls up the works. Your best chance for getting in and out quickly is to get an appointment at the beginning of the office session.

Try not to schedule your appointment on a day that is near your next menstrual period, presuming your periods are reasonably predictable. The exam will be messier and more embarrassing. It is also more difficult to obtain a satisfactory Pap smear. If your menstrual flow comes on the day of your visit, call your doctor. If your flow is light or your problem urgent, you may be asked to come in for your visit anyway.

Why do I have to wait so long in the doctor's waiting room?

At times, a doctor's waiting room appears only slightly less crowded than a bus terminal. You arrive on time, only to find a waiting room full of patients. It is frustrating to discover an office running far behind schedule when you had the courtesy to arrive on time. This problem isn't easily rectified. It is partly caused by the amount of time allotted for each patient, which is determined by how much time the average visit is expected to consume. However, the doctor cannot predict what types of problems will appear on a given day. If a series of complex difficulties arises, it will be very easy to fall behind schedule. Some patients arrive late for their appointments. This sets the schedule further behind. Certainly, many doctors underestimate the amount of time needed for the average patient and should allow more time for each appointment. If waiting is a problem, schedule your appointment early in the day. You can also call ahead on the day of your visit to see if the office is running on schedule. If the doctor is far behind, see if you can arrive later or reschedule your visit.

How often should I see the gynecologist?

Every 10 or 20 years is not sufficient! After an initial visit, women should be examined annually. If a problem warrants closer observation, the doctor will recommend more frequent visits. A family history of a gynecologic cancer may also indicate more than one exam per year. Some physicians follow up with postmenopausal women every six months, since there is an age-related increase in the incidence of most cancers.

At what age should my daughter see a gynecologist?

The standard recommendation is to consult a gynecologist at age 18 or at the onset of sexual activity, whichever comes first. We see you parents cringing. It's amazing how many parents say, "There is no way that my daughter could be sexually active!" Unless your daughter is locked in the attic, make no assumptions. Certainly if an adolescent is having a physical problem or has concerns, she should be evaluated earlier. Usually, initial discussions of menstruation, normal female development, and sexuality are addressed at home and at school. If parents feel uncomfortable discussing gynecologic topics, they should bring their teen (or preteen) to the doctor for education. This also gives your daughter an opportunity to discuss concerns she may not be willing to share at home. Assure her that she will have complete confidentiality. Do not attempt to pry information from the doctor. If your daughter wants to, she can ask the doctor to talk with you.

My daughter has a problem and refuses to see a gynecologist. What should I do?

Talk to your gynecologist. It may be that your daughter has a problem that doesn't require an office visit. Ask her if she would be more comfortable seeing a female gynecologist or a doctor other than your own. She may think that information shared with your gynecologist will be transmitted back to you. Or she may feel more at ease with your family doctor or pediatrician rather than a stranger. If the problem is beyond his or her scope, a gynecologist can be consulted.

Depending on the problem, a pelvic ultrasound scan may provide the physician with the information required to manage a problem. The ultrasound can be performed without having the patient remove her clothes (thereby diminishing the embarrassment) and is painless.

Can my family doctor do the pelvic exam?

Many physicians trained in family practice and internal medicine are able to practice basic gynecology. If comfortable with their skills, they can perform routine gynecologic exams and obtain Pap smears. They also may handle common gynecologic problems. This is reasonable as long as they are aware of their limitations. It is logical to assume, however, that a gynecologist will be more skilled in this area. For that reason, many women would rather see a gynecologist for their examinations.

Is douching a good idea?

No! For the most part, douching does more harm than good. The manufacturers of feminine hygiene products would like to convince you that these products are necessary for cleanliness. Wrong! Except when certain problems occur, the vagina maintains a normal bacterial population on its own. Douching temporarily reduces the normal bacteria, thereby giving less desirable bacteria the opportunity to dominate and increasing your risk of developing a vaginal infection. You also may develop an allergic or irritant reaction to one or more substances in the douche. Your doctor may instruct you to douche under certain circumstances, but avoid douching on a regular basis.

What do all those fancy words mean?

We often accuse lawyers of creating their own vocabulary so we will need them to interpret it for us. This is somewhat hypocritical of us, since doctors have done the same thing. After all, what is an endometrium, anyway? Here we'll explain terms used in describing the pelvic anatomy (also, see the illustrations on pages 10 and 11). Throughout the book, other terminology will be clarified. You will also find a glossary at the end.

- *Uterus:* Commonly referred to as the womb, the uterus is the reproductive organ located in a woman's pelvis that serves as an incubator for the developing fetus. It is primarily composed of muscular tissue called the myometrium. You can thank the myometrium for those wonderful labor pains and menstrual cramps. The inside of the uterus is lined with a layer of tissue referred to as the endometrium. It is predominantly composed of glandular tissue. Each month it is modified by hormones in preparation for pregnancy. If pregnancy does not occur, the endometrium is shed, creating the menstrual period.

- *Cervix:* The portion of the uterus that protrudes into the vagina, the cervix is commonly referred to as the opening of the uterus.

- *Ovary:* The ovaries are the female glands containing the eggs necessary for reproduction. The eggs reside in structures called follicles, which also produce the female hormones estrogen and progesterone.

- *Fallopian tubes:* These tubular structures transmit the egg to the uterus from the ovaries. There is an ovary and a fallopian tube on each side of the pelvis.

- *Vagina:* The vagina is a tubular canal connecting the outside of the body and the uterus. It allows for penetration by the penis so that sperm can be deposited and sent on their journey toward the egg. Most people are familiar with the term *vagina*, but we never make assumptions about this. We still recall a teenager who decided to name her newborn daughter Vagina (not Virginia). On her way to the delivery suite, she overheard the term and liked the sound of it. We can only hope she changed her mind, once enlightened about its meaning.

- *Vulva:* The region immediately external to the vagina, the vulva includes small inner folds referred to as the labia minora and larger outer folds referred to as the labia majora, which are covered with pubic hair. These are also called the inner and outer "lips" of the vagina.

- *Bladder:* Similar to a water balloon, the bladder is a structure that serves as a holding station for urine until you're ready to void it. (At least you hope it waits until you're ready.) It is located immediately in front of the uterus. The ureters are the tubes that bring urine to the bladder from the kidneys. The urethra is the tube that carries urine outside the body from the bladder. Its opening is located directly above the vagina.

- *Clitoris:* This small, protuberant structure is located between the uppermost reaches of the labia minora. It is directly above the urethral and vaginal openings. In most women, this is the genital structure most associated with generating sexual pleasure (sure, now we have your attention).

What is the doctor doing down there during the examination?

Many women don't have a clear understanding of what goes on during the pelvic exam. However, one thing is crystal clear. When someone is examining that part of your body, any amount of time is too long. What takes so long?

First, the doctor will inspect the external genitalia. They include the vulvar lips, clitoris, and the opening of the vagina (referred to medically as the vestibule). The opening of the urethra (referred to as the urethral meatus) and the perianal region are also examined (see the nearby illustration). Any unusual change in color, thickness, or texture of the skin in these areas is noted. The doctor also searches for skin lesions such as warts, cysts, and ulcerations.

A speculum is then inserted into the vagina. Opinions concerning this instrument range from "uncomfortable" to "instrument of torture." The speculum is a long, narrow device inserted into the vagina in a closed position and then opened to allow the doctor to see the vagina and cervix. Speculums are available in a variety of sizes. Your doctor should be able to find one that allows a clear view without making the procedure too uncomfortable. The amount of discomfort you feel depends on how tightly your pelvic musculature contracts around the speculum. Your natural reflex is to tighten your muscles. However, you can learn to relax them. These muscles are related to those that control voiding. Relax them as if you are ready to void urine (don't worry, you won't actually have an accident). Also think about relaxing your buttock

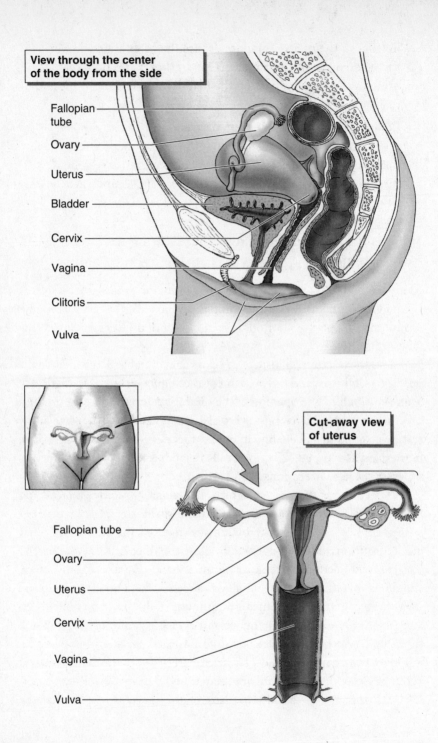

View through the center of the body from the side

Fallopian tube

Ovary

Uterus

Bladder

Cervix

Vagina

Clitoris

Vulva

Cut-away view of uterus

Fallopian tube

Ovary

Uterus

Cervix

Vagina

Vulva

ASK YOUR GYNECOLOGIST

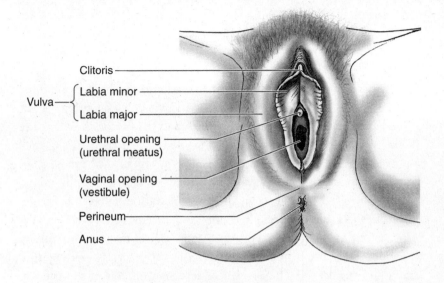

Clitoris

Vulva { Labia minor

Labia major

Urethral opening
(urethral meatus)

Vaginal opening
(vestibule)

Perineum

Anus

muscles. When you tighten your pelvic muscles, your bottom will actually start to rise. Concentrate on relaxing your bottom, and the exam will be easier. Take slow, deep breaths, exhaling completely, to relax yourself. The typical speculum feels as if it just emerged from a refrigerator. You can suggest that warming it might be in order. At this point, the doctor obtains a Pap smear (see the next question). Finally, as the speculum is removed, the vagina is evaluated for abnormalities.

Looking through the speculum, the doctor can see only the vagina and cervix, but cannot gain information regarding the rest of the uterus, the fallopian tubes, or the ovaries. Therefore, he or she will perform a manual examination, placing one or two fingers into the vagina, while placing the other hand on your lower abdomen. Using mild to moderate pressure, the doctor can feel the size, shape, and mobility of the internal organs. If you momentarily feel pain during the exam, do not misinterpret that as representing a problem. The ovaries do not like being pushed around. Once again, relaxation is of the utmost importance. Without it, the exam is more uncomfortable, and the doctor cannot get the necessary information. The doctor may also perform a rectal or recto-vaginal (one finger in the rectum and one in the vagina) exam. The structures in the posterior part of the pelvis are often assessed better through the rectum. A rectal exam should be performed on women over age 50 as a screening for rectal cancer.

What is a Pap smear?

The Papanicolaou (named after the man who introduced the technique) or "Pap" smear is a procedure whereby the gynecologist gathers cervical cells and places them on a slide for analysis. He or she takes the specimen while the speculum is open inside the vagina. A brush, small spatula, or cotton-tipped applicator is used to obtain it. In most cases the procedure is not painful, although it may feel unusual. If it is painful or uncomfortable, take solace in knowing that it doesn't take long to acquire the specimen. A specially trained technician (referred to as a cytologist) or physician (referred to as a pathologist) analyzes the cells on the slide. They use a microscope to find precancerous or cancerous changes of the cervix. The Pap smear screens women for cervical cancer only. Often women harbor the incorrect notion that the Pap smear is used to detect all types of malignancies. It does not reveal endometrial, ovarian, or vulvar cancer. A separate smear of the vagina is used to detect vaginal cancer. This procedure is not typical, since vaginal cancer is relatively uncommon.

Didn't I hear that Pap smears aren't accurate?

Throughout the years, network television has aired news segments depicting the inaccuracies of various diagnostic medical techniques. However, by focusing on the relatively small percentage of failures, these stories create a devastating misimpression. The Pap smear is a very valuable tool in the screening of cervical cancer and has been immensely successful in reducing mortality from this cancer. False negative rates do run as high as 20 percent, meaning that there is a one in five chance that an abnormality may be missed on a single Pap smear. That sounds scary, but the statistic is misleading. First, assuming you are examined annually, if an abnormality is not detected on an initial Pap smear, it is still extremely likely that it will be discovered on subsequent smears, while it is still in the precancerous state. At this stage, the condition is still readily treatable with a variety of conservative techniques. Second, current methods have improved the accuracy of

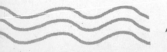

Pap smears tremendously. New technologies that use a computer to screen Pap smears (PAPNET, AutoPap) and a new method of collecting cells for the Pap test (ThinPrep Pap Test) may improve the accuracy even further. It is also fortunate that cervical cancer usually develops slowly.

What is a mammogram?

A mammogram is an x-ray of the breasts. A technician places each breast between two plates and takes a picture. A radiologist interprets the films, looking for densities within the breast tissue that could represent cancer. The size and shape of visible nodules are evaluated to determine whether they might be cancerous. Other factors taken into consideration include the sharpness of the margins (the edges or borders of the nodules) and any associated small calcium deposits. A small nodule with a regular shape, smooth margins, and no calcium deposits suggests a benign (noncancerous) density, such as a cyst. Scattered, large calcifications are fairly common and are usually benign. An enlarging nodule that is irregular and has indistinct margins suggests cancer. Clustered calcium deposits are also suspicious. In these situations, the radiologist recommends a breast biopsy (a tissue sample).

Are mammograms painful?

The answer definitely depends on whom you ask. Most women find mammography somewhat uncomfortable, but tolerable. A small number of women find mammography painful. Usually these women have cysts in their breasts (a cyst is simply a fluid-filled gland). (See chapter 12.) However, regular mammograms are particularly important for women with fibrocystic breasts because they are more difficult to examine, since they are "lumpier," making the detection of cancer more difficult.

Mammograms will also be more uncomfortable when performed shortly before the period begins. Cystic areas in the breast are more prominent at this time, which makes the interpretation of the mammogram more difficult. Schedule your mammogram early in your menstrual cycle (right after your period), and both you and your radiologist will be happier.

If you are menopausal, mammograms will be more uncomfortable if you are using hormone replacement therapy. Don't misinterpret the discomfort as a sign of a problem. If the pain is intolerable, discuss the situation with your gynecologist. He or she may be able to adjust your hormone regimen to remedy the problem.

The amount of discomfort associated with the mammogram also varies according to the technician. Often technicians are blamed for a painful mammogram. Their task is difficult. If they squeeze the breast too hard, they cause pain. If they don't squeeze it hard enough, the quality of the study is compromised.

Aren't mammograms dangerous?

Although mammograms involve a small exposure to radiation, it is a low dose. You are actually exposed to a similar dose of radiation from the environment each year. Studies do not demonstrate an adverse effect from this low dose of radiation. If there is any risk, it certainly is small. With the high incidence of breast cancer, there is no doubt that the benefits outweigh the risks.

How reliable are mammograms?

The quality of radiologic equipment used for mammograms varies. Studies have also shown that radiologists interpret the same films differently. Because of these variables, it is important to go to a facility with state-of-the-art equipment that employs radiologists with a long track record of interpreting mammograms reliably. Your gynecologist, who is the doctor primarily responsible for breast cancer screening, can recommend a facility that provides reliable results. Make sure the facility is accredited by the American College of Radiology.

The value of mammography for women over age 50 is not questioned. In this age group, approximately 90 percent of breast cancers are detected through this procedure. Early detection results in a 30 percent decrease in mortality (deaths from the cancer). Women over 50 should undergo mammograms annually.

The benefits of mammography for women under age 50 is a controversial issue. Because breast tissue in younger women is denser, it is more difficult to spot a cancer on the films. More cancers are missed.

Another concern is that breast cancer in young women often behaves aggressively. Therefore, detecting it at an earlier stage may not improve survival rates. Recent studies suggest, however, that regular screening does reduce the number of deaths due to breast cancer. Current recommendations for this age group suggest taking an initial mammogram between ages 35 and 40, followed by another every one to two years. If a woman has a close relative who developed breast cancer premenopausally, she should have annual mammograms.

Interpretation of mammographic abnormalities is not an exact science. The radiologist cannot always be certain whether a finding is benign or cancerous. Breast ultrasound (see the next question) may help determine the nature of an abnormality. A new test, called Miraluma (you have to love the name — it sounds like a Greek goddess), can also help diagnose cancer when the mammogram offers unclear information. The test uses a trace amount of radioactive isotope that temporarily accumulates in cancerous areas. These areas show up as "hot spots" on a breast image produced by a special camera. The Miraluma test may be particularly helpful for women who have dense breast tissue, breast implants, or scars from previous surgery, all of which lessen the clarity of mammograms.

Three-dimensional MRI (magnetic resonance imaging) is another promising technique for the detection of breast tumors, since the resulting images can make it possible to distinguish between abnormal (cancerous) and normal breast tissue better than images from standard mammography. However, high cost and the fact that the procedure is not available everywhere limit its use as a screening tool. Digital mammography (using computer-aided technology) and laser mammography (using a laser scanner) are also on the horizon and should improve the diagnostic accuracy of mammography.

Why do I have to get a breast ultrasound?

Although mammography effectively reveals a breast nodule or mass, it cannot show whether it is solid or cystic. Breast ultrasound provides this information. A fluid-filled structure is considered cystic and therefore benign. The risk of cancer is greater with a solid mass. It is usually biopsied. The breast ultrasound does not replace the mammogram, but rather gives additional information. If your mammogram is normal, a breast ultrasound is not necessary.

How can I lose this weight?

You didn't have this question in mind when you made your appointment. Unfortunately, the nurse had the gall to weigh you before you entered the exam room. How could you possibly have gained another ten pounds? You haven't been eating any differently. This isn't fair!

Although weight control is seldom related to gynecologic disorders, invariably our patients ask about it. Whether you have struggled with weight control or passively watched your weight spiral upward, you are not alone. Currently, more Americans are overweight than at a normal weight. How much weight is too much? As a rule, a woman who is five feet tall should weigh 100 pounds. You can then add 5 pounds for every inch above five feet, plus or minus 10 percent. If you're not sure, your doctor can refer to a chart that indicates a normal range of weight for your height. If you are more than 20 percent overweight, the doctor may even use that hideous term, *obese*. Weight gain occurs when you consume more energy (as food) than you burn. Although weight problems can result from certain medical conditions such as hypothyroidism or from taking certain medications, usually heredity, eating habits, and overall lifestyle dictate your weight.

Tackling a weight problem is a difficult endeavor. There are no shortcuts, no instant cures for the problem. The most sensible approach is a gradual change to a low-fat, healthful diet and increased exercise. Fad diets that severely restrict calories are not the answer. When these diets are discontinued, weight rebounds, often shooting higher than before. Modest reduction in calories (300 to 500 per day) is reasonable and usually occurs naturally with a change to a low-fat diet rich in fruits, grains, pasta, and vegetables. Total fat intake should be less than 30 percent of total calories. Especially avoid saturated fats — your heart and arteries will thank you later. Try the following suggestions to help in losing weight:

- Avoid alcohol, which contains "empty calories" with no nutritional value.

- Drink plenty of water — up to eight glasses of it every day (unless you must restrict fluids for other health reasons).
- Avoid second helpings.
- If you are hungry between meals, choose a healthful snack (fruit) over an unhealthful one (ice cream, potato chips).
- Don't eat while reading or watching television.
- Try not to eat for the wrong reasons (to cope with boredom, stress, depression).
- Eat out less often — and when you do eat out, be selective in choosing your food.
- Perhaps most important, increase your exercise.

Exercise does not have to be tedious and boring. Choose an activity that you enjoy, such as tennis, golf, swimming, or dancing. Even 30 minutes of brisk walking every day will make a difference. We can hear you saying, "I don't have the time to exercise." Do you have time to read or watch television? If so, you have the time to exercise. Both of these activities can be done while exercising. Buy a treadmill or exercise bike, and put it in front of the television.

"I have arthritis" (or bursitis, or tendinitis — insert your own "itis") "so I can't exercise." Nice try, but we're not buying it. Usually some form of exercise can be adapted to accommodate your medical condition. If you have arthritis, you will probably enjoy working out in a swimming pool (pool aerobics are great) because being suspended in water takes the weight off your joints.

If you can make this commitment to a lifestyle change, you will not only lose the pounds, but also keep them off.

What if I have pain?

There is nothing worse than pain! Even those who avoid the doctor's office for almost any reason relent when pain occurs. It is one of the more common reasons for a woman to see her gynecologist. Any pain in the lower abdomen or pelvic region is assumed to be related to the "female organs." Although this may indeed be the case, there are multiple causes of pain.

You should see a doctor if your pain is severe, worsening, recurrent, or disruptive to your daily life. Changes in your bowel function, bladder function, or menstrual cycle, or a rise in your temperature to above 100 degrees, should also prompt you to seek help. Initial evaluation can be made by your primary care doctor or your gynecologist. It is probably most appropriate to see your primary care doctor if the pain is in the middle or upper abdomen or associated with gastrointestinal symptoms (nausea, vomiting, diarrhea, constipation). Your gynecologist can evaluate unexplained pain in the lower abdomen. Before seeing the doctor, try to characterize your pain. How long does it last? Is it constant or intermittent? How frequently does it occur? Is it sharp or dull? Does it occur at a particular time of your menstrual cycle? This information will help your doctor evaluate your condition.

Pain accompanied by nausea and vomiting or change in bowel function is usually gastrointestinal in origin. Upper abdominal pain can result from problems involving the stomach (gastritis, ulcers, reflux esophagitis), pancreas, liver, and gallbladder. Lower abdominal pain can be caused by colitis, irritable bowel disease, diverticulitis, or appendicitis. Cancer within the abdomen can cause pain, so do not ignore persistent discomfort. If one of these conditions is suspected, your doctor may consult with either a surgeon (in the case of appendicitis or other surgical conditions) or a gastroenterologist (for conditions that do not require surgery).

Pain associated with bladder symptoms, such as frequency and urgency of urination, painful urination, or bloody urine, is usually urologic in origin. Possible causes include infection of the bladder or kidneys, "kidney stones," cancer, and interstitial cystitis. These are explored in chapter 14.

Muscle strain or spasm can also produce pain in the lower abdomen or pelvis. This may occur because of weakness in or injury to the abdominal, back, or pelvic floor muscles. Muscle spasm may also result from disc disease or arthritis in the spine. Damage to nerves emerging from the lower back or coursing through the pelvis may also cause pelvic pain.

Pelvic pain can also arise from many gynecologic conditions. We'll

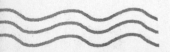

only briefly describe them here because most are explored in other chapters:

- *Infections:* Pelvic inflammatory disease is an infection of the uterus, fallopian tubes, and ovaries. Most cases come from sexually transmitted organisms. Common symptoms include lower abdominal or pelvic pain, fever, and discharge. Pain limited to the vagina or vulva may be caused by herpes or vaginitis. Pelvic infections are addressed in chapter 5.

- *Complications of pregnancy:* Miscarriage and ectopic pregnancy (a pregnancy located outside the uterus, usually in a fallopian tube) may cause pain. If you have missed your usual menstrual period and develop pain, you should be evaluated promptly. Refer to chapter 7 for more information about these conditions. Your doctor can easily exclude complications of pregnancy by obtaining a blood pregnancy test (referred to as HCG or B-HCG).

- *Ovarian cysts and tumors:* When the ovary develops a cyst or growth, it enlarges. You may sense a fullness in the pelvic region, or a dull ache. If a cyst ruptures, you may experience sharp pain that goes away within a day or two. An enlarged ovary may also twist and turn, causing intermittent pain. Ovarian cysts are common, and most disappear spontaneously. However, large or persistent cysts may require surgery. Benign (noncancerous) tumors and ovarian cancer may also cause pelvic pain. Ovarian cysts and tumors are reviewed in chapter 10.

- *Uterine conditions:* Uterine fibroids are benign smooth-muscle tumors that develop within the wall of the uterus. It is uncommon for fibroids to cause pain, although they may do so if they markedly enlarge and press on other organs or outgrow their blood supply and undergo a process called degeneration. Adenomyosis is a condition in which the inside lining of the uterus (endometrium) "grows" into the muscular wall of the uterus (myometrium). Adenomyosis causes menstrual cramps and heavy menstrual flow, worsening in a woman's late thirties or forties. Uterine cancer may cause pelvic pain, although this is often a late symptom; abnormal bleeding would usually signal the cancer's presence much earlier. We discuss fibroids and adenomyosis in chapter 9.

- *Endometriosis:* Endometriosis is a condition in which endometrial tissue (normally found lining the inside of the uterus) is located outside the uterus. It may cause painful menstrual cramps, chronic pelvic pain, or painful intercourse. We will discuss endometriosis and its related problems in chapter 8.

- *Adhesions:* Adhesions (scar tissue) can form as a result of anything that causes inflammation in the pelvic region, including pelvic infections, endometriosis, and prior surgical procedures. Pain from adhesions is usually chronic in nature and often unassociated with other symptoms.

- *Functional pain:* You can have "functional" pain that does not come from disease. This seems counterintuitive. If everything is normal, why is there pain? Painful menstrual cramps (dysmenorrhea) may occur without other disease. This is particularly true if you have always had painful periods. Some women will get recurrent midcycle pain associated with ovulation. These and other menstrual disorders are discussed in chapter 2.

You can see from this list (if you're not totally confused by now) that there are myriad potential causes for pain in the lower abdomen. Sometimes the source of pain is obvious. It can, however, be very perplexing. Your doctor may have to approach the problem one step at a time, gradually eliminating causes until he or she correctly diagnoses the conditions. The evaluation begins by taking down a careful history and making an examination. If the source of your pain is not obvious, the doctor will order laboratory tests such as bloodwork, urine studies, or imaging studies to gain more information. These might include any of the following:

- *Pelvic ultrasound:* This imaging scan uses sound waves (no radiation) to generate a picture of the pelvic organs. Ovarian cysts and tumors, fibroids, pregnancy (normal and abnormal), pelvic abscesses, and large kidney stones can all be revealed by ultrasound.

- *Computed tomography (CT or CAT scan):* This type of x-ray produces images of the internal organs. This information can help the doctor diagnose benign and malignant tumors as well as certain types of inflammatory conditions.

- *Magnetic resonance imaging (MRI):* This method of viewing the internal organs uses a magnetic field. Certain types of abnormalities can be seen more easily or clearly with MRI.

- *Barium enema:* Barium is put into the colon through the rectum. This white material allows clear pictures of the lower bowel to be obtained by x-ray. If there is need to evaluate the upper intestinal tract, barium can be swallowed before the x-ray is taken.

- *Intravenous pyelogram (IVP):* In this procedure, dye is injected into a vein, the kidneys excrete the dye into the urinary tract, and x-rays are taken, providing good images of the kidneys, ureters, and bladder.

Telescopic instruments may be used for further examination if the source of pain is still unclear. The gastrointestinal tract can be evaluated by either endoscopy (placing a flexible telescopic instrument down the throat) or colonoscopy (you guessed it — through the rectum). Cystoscopy enables a urologist to look into the bladder. Gynecologists use either a hysteroscope to look into the uterus without making an incision or a laparoscope to look into the abdomen through a tiny incision near your navel. Sometimes these procedures are done in an office setting, and other times they are performed as outpatient surgery. A local anesthetic, intravenous sedation, or general anesthesia may be used for these procedures.

Treatment of pain varies according to its source, but is likely to include medications called analgesics. You are already familiar with the more common ones, such as acetaminophen (Tylenol) and ibuprofen (Motrin, Advil). More intense pain is treated with drugs containing narcotics. These will be more effective at relieving pain but generally have more side effects, such as nausea and drowsiness. They should not be taken if you must be alert for any reason, especially if you will need to drive a car or operate machinery. (Then again, if you're in that much pain, you probably should be at home resting.)

Chronic pain is particularly distressing. Not all pain can be eradicated. Chronic pain syndrome may ensue, which is difficult to cope with physically and emotionally. Other medications may be added to analgesics to treat chronic pain. Antidepressants have been used successfully for patients with chronic pain. They act on pain impulses at a different location than analgesics do, and the two can be used together. Other methods, such as biofeedback, relaxation techniques, physical therapy, and transcutaneous electrical nerve stimulation (TENS, which creates tiny electrical nerve impulses at the affected site to block pain impulses), may also be effective. Often a multidisciplinary approach that involves several doctors and therapists is the best answer for patients with chronic pain syndrome. Emotional support is often required. A competent therapist may be a critical resource in coping with the psychological struggles associated with chronic pain.

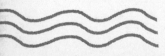

2 The Menstrual Cycle: What's Normal, What's Not

What's a normal cycle?

Many concerns about menstruation are based on a misunderstanding of the normal menstrual cycle. Any variation in the cycle may be interpreted as abnormal and worrisome. Explaining the menstrual cycle is only slightly easier than outlining Einstein's theory of relativity, but let's try.

The menstrual cycle is composed of two phases. It begins with the follicular phase. Located in the ovaries, follicles are small fluid-filled structures that contain an egg. The cycle begins when one of the follicles matures, generally over the course of two weeks, and produces estrogen. Estrogen stimulates the endometrium (the lining of the uterus), causing it to thicken. When follicular maturation is complete, the egg is released to embark on its journey down the fallopian tube. This is referred to as ovulation. After ovulation, the second phase of the menstrual cycle, called the luteal phase, begins. The follicular structure (now referred to as the corpus luteum) continues to produce estrogen. It also produces a second hormone called progesterone. Progesterone alters the endometrium, preparing it for implantation of a fertilized egg. If the egg is not fertilized, the ovary stops producing the female hormones. Without hormonal support, the endometrium is shed as a menstrual flow, commonly known as the period. The cycle begins again as another follicle matures. (For an illustration of the female reproductive system, see page 24.)

The average length of a complete cycle is four weeks. It is, however, common for the cycle to vary in length from three to five weeks. It is most variable near the time of the first menstrual period and then again

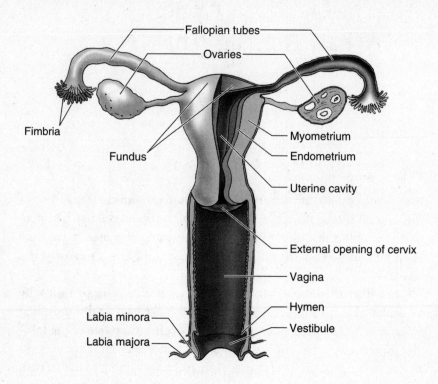

as menopause approaches. Some women never achieve a regular cycle. If your cycle varies between three to eight weeks, and your menstrual flow lasts for less than one week, don't worry about it. If you are bleeding more frequently than every three weeks or have not had a menstrual period in eight weeks, you should contact your gynecologist. You are probably no longer having ovulatory cycles, and hormonal intervention may be necessary.

Why do I get pain in the middle of my cycle?

You're in the supermarket. You're just about to reach for the frozen lasagna, when suddenly a pain appears out of nowhere. After a few hours it subsides, but you're still wondering, "What was that?" If it oc-

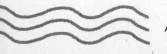

curred in the middle of your cycle, you just experienced mittelschmerz. Discomfort is often felt in the pelvis during ovulation. Usually the pain is transient, but it can persist for a day or two. When severe, it is termed mittelschmerz (from the German words meaning "middle pain"). If you menstruate two weeks after the pain occurs, no special investigation is necessary. If the pain is severe, take acetaminophen (Tylenol or a generic equivalent). If the pain is disabling and you do not wish to become pregnant, consider asking your gynecologist to prescribe oral contraceptives (the birth control pill). By inhibiting ovulation, they will solve your problem.

I'm late for my period. Am I pregnant?

This question is associated with the most anxious moments in one's life. "I'm late for my period . . . aaaah . . . help!" Often, though, a missed period does not indicate pregnancy. The menstrual cycle may simply be "out of sync." In this situation, the body's normal signals that control ovarian function have become confused. Ovulation doesn't occur, and the ovary fails to produce progesterone. Without progesterone, the endometrium will not be shed, and thus no period occurs.

If your pregnancy test is negative, your doctor can prescribe a short course of progesterone to induce the menstrual flow. It is not prudent to wait longer than two to three months before beginning progesterone. During the time you are not ovulating, the ovary continues to produce estrogen, stimulating the endometrium and causing it to thicken. Eventually, the endometrium will break down, causing heavy or erratic bleeding.

I get my period only two or three times during the year. Is that OK?

This may sound great. No bleeding, and think of all the savings on pads and tampons. Heck, while you're at it, why can't you get rid of periods altogether? Unfortunately, this is not in your best interest.

Infrequent menses (called oligomenorrhea) and totally absent menses (amenorrhea) usually mean that you are not ovulating on a regular basis. Both conditions can produce heavy or erratic bleeding and eventually increase your risk for developing endometrial cancer.

There are numerous reasons for skipping a menstrual period. Some are quite simple, such as stress or anxiety. Abrupt weight gain or loss and vigorous exercise are also culprits. Certain medications alter your cycle by interfering with the female hormones. Various medical disorders can upset your cycle. The most common is thyroid disease.

If your menstrual periods are infrequent, talk to your gynecologist. Usually, no distressing problem is found. Your gynecologist will recommend either progesterone or oral contraceptives to improve your hormonal balance, decreasing the chance of experiencing erratic bleeding.

I get terrible cramps with my period. What's wrong?

Cramps are induced by the release of substances called prostaglandins from the endometrium (the inner lining of the uterus), causing contractions in the muscular wall of the uterus. The wall of the intestines also has a muscular layer, which may also be affected by the prostaglandins. Therefore, nausea and loose bowel movements often accompany uterine cramps. Nonprescription medications that offer relief by combating prostaglandins include ibuprofen (Advil, Nuprin, Medipren, and Motrin), naproxen sodium (Aleve), and ketoprofen (Orudis, Actron). Oral contraceptives, which thin the endometrium, are also used. Menses then become lighter and less painful.

If your menses have only recently became painful, you may have an underlying disorder. A common offender is endometriosis, a condition in which endometrial tissue is found outside the uterus. Endometriosis is particularly suspected if the pain starts during the days leading up to your menses. (See chapter 8 for more information.) Other causes for pain include adenomyosis, pelvic infection, uterine polyps, and fibroids. These are described extensively in other chapters.

Inform your gynecologist if your menstrual periods are unusually painful. He or she may want to obtain more information through pelvic ultrasound or cultures. If no obvious source for your pain is found, the doctor will recommend antiprostaglandins or oral contraceptives. If your pain is severe, laparoscopy or hysteroscopy may be indicated. Laparoscopy is a surgical procedure that allows the doctor to view the internal pelvic organs through a telescopic instrument inserted into the abdomen. Hysteroscopy is a telescopic look at the inside of the uterus that is done by way of the vagina, without making an incision.

When my period comes, I flood. Is that normal?

Assessing your bleeding can be surprisingly difficult. What one person considers heavy may be normal to another. If you are saturating maxi pads every hour or two, your bleeding is unusually heavy. Occasionally, a woman has a history of heavy menstrual periods her entire life. This condition may be normal, but if you have it, you should be checked to make sure that you don't have a problem with blood clotting.

If your menstrual flow is becoming progressively heavier, it is abnormal. Don't let this persist without investigation. What seems to be a mere nuisance now could become a life-threatening hemorrhage in the future. If the timing of your period is erratic, your problem may relate to abnormal production of the female hormones. In this case, artificially regulating your cycle corrects the problem. However, if your cycle appears to be regular, the heavier flow is probably caused by an intrinsic disorder of the uterus, such as fibroids, polyps, and adenomyosis. Your doctor will probably want a pelvic ultrasound scan to give a clearer picture of your pelvic organs. An endometrial biopsy, D&C (dilation and curettage, in which the endometrium is scraped and the sample is evaluated under a microscope), or hysteroscopy may be needed. These are discussed extensively in chapter 9.

If your flow is heavy, drink more fluids than usual to ward off dizziness. Also take an iron supplement to prevent anemia. Iron often irritates the gastrointestinal system, resulting in constipation or diarrhea. Your doctor can recommend a brand of iron that is less likely to produce these effects.

What does it mean when I get clots during my period?

Blood clots during menstrual flow can be startling. Because of their striking appearance, it can be easy to assume that they mean that something is wrong. Actually, blood clots do not reflect a specific problem. If blood remains inside the uterus long enough, it will clot. However, copious, large clots reflect heavy bleeding and should be brought to the attention of your doctor.

Is bleeding between my periods normal?

Bleeding between periods is referred to as intermenstrual bleeding. When you ovulate, you get a hormonal surge, and you may have light bleeding for a day or two. Mark on your calendar the day the bleeding occurred, and wait for your next menstrual period. If your menses follows the bleeding episode by two weeks, assume it is normal.

Intermenstrual bleeding that occurs at other times in the cycle is not acceptable. The abnormal bleeding may be caused by a hormonal variation. However, as you advance in age, other conditions such as fibroids, polyps, and even cancer become possibilities. Other less likely culprits include cervical or vaginal lesions, endometriosis, uterine infection, and ovarian disorders. Your doctor can readily eliminate vaginal or cervical causes for the bleeding if these structures appear normal on your speculum examination and if your Pap smear is normal.

If you are younger than age 35 and your exam is normal, no further evaluation is necessary. If bleeding persists over several months, your cycle can be regulated artificially to correct the problem. If it does not respond to hormonal manipulation, additional studies should be undertaken. These may include pelvic ultrasound, endometrial biopsy, D&C, and hysteroscopy.

Over the age of 35 (some doctors say age 40), intermenstrual bleeding may indicate precancerous and cancerous uterine conditions. Although this is the least likely root of your problem, it is the most critical to diagnose. Evaluation of the endometrium with an endometrial biopsy, D&C, or hysteroscopy is mandatory. Pelvic ultrasound is also helpful. If no underlying condition is discovered, the doctor will attempt hormonal regulation with either progestational agents or oral contraceptives.

What can I do if I have PMS?

Your son has that quizzical look that says, "Has Mom lost her mind? All I did was spill my milk, and she went ballistic." Your husband remarks, "Is it that time of the month already?" Every month you get tense and irritable before your period. In all likelihood, you have premenstrual syndrome. Premenstrual syndrome (PMS) encompasses a wide range of

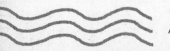

physical and emotional symptoms that repetitively occur during the week or two immediately preceding your menses. Common physical symptoms include breast tenderness, fluid retention, bloating, and fatigue. Appetite changes, food cravings, headaches, nausea, constipation, dizziness, clumsiness, and a host of other physical symptoms have also been linked to PMS. Common emotional symptoms include mood swings, irritability, anxiety, and depression. You don't have to experience all of these symptoms to have PMS, but the symptoms must occur only premenstrually. If you are not sure, keep a diary to establish the timing of your symptoms.

Despite many claims, nobody really understands the cause of PMS. Many assume that the symptoms are produced by alterations in the levels of the female hormones estrogen and progesterone. Since the disorder appears in women only between the onset of menstruation and menopause, this theory appears logical. However, scientific studies have established that hormone levels are normal in patients with PMS. It may be that certain individuals are more sensitive to various hormonal effects in certain areas of the body. Premenstrual mood and anxiety disorders are likely created by alterations in chemicals produced in the brain that are referred to as neurotransmitters.

The physical symptoms of PMS are easier to control than the emotional ones. Swelling in the hands or feet is caused by fluid retention. Eliminating salt from your diet is an initial step to approaching this problem. A mild diuretic (a "water pill"), a medication that helps your kidneys excrete excess fluid, can be prescribed. Bloating reflects increased intestinal gas. It may be associated with constipation. Often a change in diet will help reduce these symptoms. Avoid foods that increase gas production (beans, cabbage, broccoli, carbonated beverages), and increase your fiber intake. Over-the-counter preparations containing simethicone (Mylicon or Gas X) dissipate gas in your bowel, thereby increasing comfort. Breast tenderness may decrease if fluid retention is eliminated. Decreasing caffeine consumption (coffee, tea, colas, chocolate) and taking supplemental vitamin E (400 to 800 international units, or IU, per day) appear to help some women, although medical evidence of their benefit is scanty (see pages 154–55). Nonprescription pain relievers containing acetaminophen (Tylenol) or ibuprofen (Advil, Nuprin, Motrin) should also be considered. If your breast tenderness is particularly severe, special medications can be prescribed. However, they all have potential side effects that may be undesirable. Your doctor can review these with you if the preceding suggestions are not helpful. Eating five or six small meals daily, high in complex carbohydrates (vegetables, whole grains, legumes) and low in simple carbohydrates (refined sugar, soft drinks), can help you keep food cravings in check.

The emotional symptoms associated with PMS are more difficult to manage. Many solutions have been touted as successful, only to fall short under closer scrutiny. Two extensively utilized treatments are progesterone and vitamin B_6. Unfortunately, in well-designed studies, these do not appear to be more effective than a placebo (a pill that contains no medication). One has to be careful in attributing therapeutic value to a treatment for PMS because there is a very high placebo effect. If you are really convinced that something should help you, there is a good chance it will, but the positive effects won't last. Another promising treatment, the amino acid L-tryptophan, was discontinued when it was found to cause a blood disorder.

So where does this leave us? Here are some suggestions. First, modify your diet to reduce intake of caffeine, salt, sugar, and alcohol. All of these in one way or another can affect your mood. Next, start a vigorous exercise program. Exercise not only strengthens the body but also relieves tension and elevates mood. Try to schedule stressful activities earlier in your cycle. Incorporate stress reduction into your daily routine. This might include listening to or playing music, going for a walk, meditating, or listening to relaxation tapes. You're thinking, "They have to be crazy. I barely have enough time to breathe, and they want me to relax." It may be difficult, but sit down with your family and discuss ways to make time for yourself.

If PMS interferes significantly with your ability to function either at home or work, then more aggressive treatment is required. Antianxiety and antidepressant medications may be effective. Ask your doctor if one is appropriate for you.

We can't leave this issue without rendering an opinion on over-the-

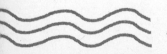

counter PMS preparations (Midol PMS, Premsyn PMS, Pamprin). Most of these contain acetaminophen (as does Tylenol), a mild diuretic, and an antihistamine that has sedative effects. You may gain some relief with these products (particularly if you *really* think they will help). However, they are mild and are not likely to be successful with severe PMS. Combination herbal and vitamin remedies (PMS Herbal, Pre-Menses P.M.S., PMS Nutritional System) contain herbs such as black cohosh and dong quai and megadoses of vitamins. Although they may alleviate some symptoms, there is not enough scientific evidence proving their efficacy and safety to recommend their use. In fact, vitamin B_6, which is found in these preparations, can cause nerve damage in doses higher than 200 milligrams. A drink mix called PMS Escape attempts to relieve food cravings and moodiness by increasing serotonin levels. It contains 47 grams of carbohydrates (188 calories) and vitamins. Although there is evidence that carbohydrates can boost serotonin levels (and thereby elevate mood), two cups of cereal or pasta will provide the same amount of carbohydrates. Feminine hormone creams (Maxine's Feminique Balancing Cream, Femarone, Phillips Yamcon) contain hormonal extracts from yams. Homeopathic remedies (PMS Relief, Natural Phases, Medicine from Nature's PMS) contain minuscule amounts of various herbs. Once again, there is inadequate evidence to confirm their effectiveness and safety.

I always get a headache at the beginning of my period. Why?

We're talking big-time pain — throbbing headaches. They appear before or during the first few days of your period. You may be experiencing menstrual migraine headaches. Your hormone levels drop immediately before the onset of your flow. This can trigger a migraine headache. Typically, a migraine brings severe pain limited to one side of your head. Sometimes it is preceded by visual effects, such as flashing lights or partial loss of vision. Nausea and vomiting may accompany the headache. Intolerance to loud noises and bright lights is common. Migraines are more common in women than men. Common triggers for migraines include changes in humidity, changes in altitude and barometric pressure, flashing lights, loud noises, changes in sleeping habits (oversleeping), missed meals, hormone changes, and certain foods. If you're predisposed to migraines, the following foods may induce a headache:

- Bananas (more than half a banana daily)
- Beans (lima, fava, snow peas)
- Chicken livers, pâté
- Chocolate
- Citrus fruit (more than half a cup daily)
- Coffee, cola, tea (more than two cups daily)
- Figs, raisins, papayas, avocados, red plums (more than half a cup daily)
- Herring (or any food that is fermented, pickled, or marinated)
- MSG (monosodium glutamate — may be found in soy sauce, meat tenderizer, seasoned salt, Chinese food, salad bars)
- Nuts, peanut butter
- Pizza
- Processed meats (sausage, bologna, pepperoni, salami, hot dogs, bacon)
- Ripened cheeses (cheddar, Emmentaler, Stilton, Brie, Camembert)
- Sour cream (more than half a cup daily)
- Sourdough bread

Now that we've eliminated all your favorite foods, you may decide you'd rather have a headache. Actually, everyone is unique. The above list is only a guide. Keep track of your diet to see which foods trigger your migraines, and adjust your food choices accordingly.

There are a number of approaches to the treatment of migraine headaches. Some women gain adequate relief with over-the-counter or prescribed analgesics (painkillers). Sumatriptan (Imitrex) is a non-narcotic drug that is particularly good at alleviating migraine attacks. Other medications that can reduce the frequency of migraines include antidepressants, beta-blockers, and calcium channel blockers. A complete discussion of these is beyond the scope of this book, but ask your doctor about them if your headaches are frequent.

Menstrual migraines may be triggered by prostaglandins released at menstruation (see page 26). Anti-prostaglandin medications such as ibuprofen (Motrin, Advil, and others) or naproxen sodium (Anaprox, Aleve) may reduce the frequency of migraines. Estrogen fluctuations may also trigger migraines. This may be prevented by starting an estrogen supplement near the end of the cycle (between days 24 and 28 for cycles lasting 28 days). For unpredictable cycles, estrogen can be consumed when premenstrual symptoms (breast tenderness, bloating) occur. The estrogen is continued during the first few days of the menstrual flow.

If you get migraines, you should make a concerted effort to eat balanced meals at regular intervals and avoid alcohol and caffeine. Dietary triggers should be reduced at times when you seem vulnerable to migraines. Stress reduction and regular exercise are also beneficial. Biofeedback and acupuncture have been found effective in reducing migraine headache pain. If skilled therapists offer these treatments in your area, you might try them.

Additional information can be obtained by calling the National Headache Foundation (800-843-2256) or at its web site (http://www.headaches.org).

My daughter is 15 and still hasn't gotten her period. Should I be worried?

Your daughter may feel embarrassed if her friends are menstruating and she is not. It seems that they are progressing into womanhood, leaving her behind. Reassurance is all that is necessary. There is a wide variation in the onset of the first menstrual period, which is referred to as menarche. The average age of onset is 12, but up to 16 may be normal. The development of other sexual characteristics such as breast formation and pubic hair typically precedes menarche, as does the growth spurt. If these are not present by age 14, consultation with an endocrinologist or a gynecologist who specializes in endocrine disorders is a requirement. If these sexual characteristics are developing and growth is on schedule, then it is reasonable to wait until age 16 before seeing a specialist. Also, it is common for the menstrual period to be erratic in the year following menarche. If the cycle ranges anywhere from three to eight weeks apart and the duration of flow is less than a week, no action is necessary. Her cycle will likely become regular within one to two years, without treatment.

Are tampons safe?

In 1980, toxic shock syndrome was diagnosed in a number of menstruating women. Mass hysteria followed. We can understand the panic. A person could be placed in solitary confinement for a month and not come up with a name as ominous as toxic shock syndrome. What is this terrible disease? It causes fever, diffuse rash, and faintness during menstruation or shortly thereafter. Nausea, vomiting, diarrhea, cramping, disorientation, and loss of consciousness are also common. Toxic shock syndrome is caused by the release of toxins from a bacterium called *Staphylococcus aureus.* This bacterium is present in the vaginas of approximately 5 percent of all women. The disease can also be seen in men and nonmenstruating women who develop other types of infections from the bacterium. Although toxic shock syndrome can be severe, it is rare. Even at its peak, the incidence did not exceed 15 cases per 100,000 menstruating women per year. It was found to be associated with the use of superabsorbent tampons, particularly one called Rely. Women began to question the safety of tampons. After the Rely tampon was withdrawn from the market, the incidence decreased to 1 per 100,000 women each year. You should not avoid using tampons because of concern about toxic shock syndrome. It does, however, make sense to avoid superabsorbent tampons (labeled as such on the package), unless your flow is very heavy and you expect to change tampons frequently. Tampons should not be left in place for a prolonged time (greater than eight hours).

You may be concerned about injuring yourself when you insert a tampon. Don't worry: Genital injury caused by putting in or removing tampons is extremely uncommon. Virginal women may have difficulty. Using slender models of tampons with lubrication such as K-Y jelly may help in this situation. If you still have difficulty, schedule a gynecologic exam.

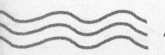

ASK YOUR GYNECOLOGIST

③ Contraception: Weighing the Alternatives

Is it possible to get pregnant the first time I have sex?

You'd be surprised how many women — particularly teens — think that multiple sexual encounters are required for conception to occur. Many times when one of us asks a woman who says she has missed her period whether she might be pregnant, she responds, "No, I only had sex once." Sometimes, once is enough. The time to think about contraception is before you achieve that level of intimacy.

What is natural family planning?

No, this doesn't mean children are grown organically. Many couples want to prevent pregnancy without using "artificial" contraceptives and instead refrain from intercourse during the time in the cycle when the chance of conception is greatest — anywhere from five days before ovulation through two days after. This is referred to as natural family planning. The key to its success is determining the day of ovulation. In most cases, ovulation will predictably occur 14 days before the next menstrual period. For example, if a woman's cycle interval (the number of days from the first day of one period to the first day of the next period) is 32 days, she ovulates on day 18 and would abstain from intercourse on days 13 through 20.

If you wish to proceed with natural family planning, you must pinpoint your day of ovulation, by charting your basal body temperature. Your doctor can provide you with a chart and instructions. In this method, you check your temperature upon awakening each morning. Your temperature rises approximately one-half degree 24 hours after ovulation. By reviewing the chart, you can determine when ovulation has occurred.

Checking your cervical mucus can also help determine the day of ovulation. Your cervix (the opening of the uterus) produces mucus that is secreted into the vagina. Before ovulation, the mucus is voluminous and has a watery texture, and when you observe this, you should refrain from intercourse. After ovulation, the mucus is reduced in amount and becomes thicker.

A high level of motivation is required to carry out successful natural family planning. Before deciding whether to use this method, you should be aware that surveys indicate a 25 percent failure rate over the course of one year.

What is barrier contraception?

You can't erect a barricade to hold off the millions of sperm attacking your egg, but you do have the benefit of barrier contraception. Barrier contraceptives include condoms, diaphragms, and spermicides. They do just what their name implies: They form a barrier between his sperm and your egg. These contraceptives function either as physical barriers (condoms and diaphragms) or chemical barriers (spermicides).

The diaphragm is a dome-shaped rubber device inserted into the vagina prior to intercourse. It is used with a spermicidal cream or jelly to enhance protection. Apply spermicide to the diaphragm, which must be inserted no more than two hours prior to intercourse. It must remain in place for at least six hours after intercourse. If you have intercourse again before six hours, place another applicator of spermicide into the vagina. Your doctor will fit you with a diaphragm of the correct size and will instruct you on proper placement. Make sure you can insert and re-move the diaphragm properly before leaving the office. If the dia-phragm fits properly, it shouldn't feel uncomfortable. Replace it every two years or if it develops holes or tears. Have the size checked if you gain or lose more than 20 pounds. Also have it rechecked after preg-nancy. When used properly, diaphragms are 85 to 90 percent effective at preventing pregnancy.

Cervical caps are smaller, dome-shaped devices that fit tightly on

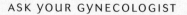

the cervix. Although more effective than the diaphragm, they are generally more difficult to use. Currently, they are not in widespread use in this country, although this may change. For more information about their availability, contact your doctor.

Condoms are available in male and female versions. They are readily available over the counter in most pharmacies. The male condom is a sheath, usually composed of latex, placed over the erect penis. Condoms should be removed before the penis is limp, to prevent leakage of semen into the vagina. Female condoms (Reality) have recently become available and appear to be effective. The female condom is composed of a polyurethane (a type of plastic) pouch with a ring at both ends. The inner ring is placed deep in the vagina while the external ring remains outside. The female condom may be less disruptive than the male condom because it may be inserted up to eight hours prior to intercourse, so you don't have to stop in the middle of foreplay to put it in. Do not use a male and a female condom at the same time.

One of the biggest advantages of condoms is protection against sexually transmitted diseases (see chapter 5). However, some male condoms are made of animal membranes that do not afford this protection. For the best defense against pregnancy and disease, use latex condoms. Condoms are approximately 90 percent effective at preventing pregnancy. Their success is increased with the addition of a spermicide.

If you are allergic to latex (as evidenced by the fact that your vagina becomes inflamed whenever you use a condom), consider trying either the female condom (Reality) or the male condom Avanti. Both are made with polyurethane instead of latex.

Is withdrawal a good method of contraception?

We're assuming you have a partner who is willing to remove his penis from the vagina prior to ejaculation. This is a huge assumption. You're asking him to stop the very activity that has brought him to the peak of arousal. If he is able to withdraw before ejaculation, it certainly decreases your chances of pregnancy. However, this method is far from foolproof. A small amount of semen emanates from the penis prior to ejaculation, which may be sufficient for conception. If there is sudden ejaculation, even larger amounts of semen will be deposited into the vagina prior to his withdrawal. If you really want to avoid becoming pregnant, don't rely on withdrawal.

How good are over-the-counter foams and inserts?

Spermicides encompass creams, foams, jellies, and vaginal suppositories containing a chemical that kills sperm. They are easier to use than physical barriers, but are less effective. Spermicides are 70 to 80 percent successful at preventing pregnancy. This means you have a one in five chance of becoming pregnant over the course of one year. Spermicides are most reliable when used with a condom or diaphragm. Allergic or irritant reactions sometimes occur with spermicides. If you note severe vaginal burning or itching, discontinue using them.

Why should I take the birth control pill?

Birth control pills, also referred to as oral contraceptives or "the pill," are extremely effective. When used properly, their success rate is over 99 percent. Birth control pills work by inhibiting ovulation. They are easier to use and more convenient than barrier methods of contraception. Their contraceptive effect is easily reversible when you want to conceive. Modern pills, which contain lower doses of hormones than older versions, are usually tolerated quite well.

In addition, the pill has numerous health benefits. Menstrual cycles are very regular on oral contraceptives and flow will usually be lighter. The risk of iron deficiency anemia is reduced. Women with painful periods usually have fewer cramps while on the pill. The pill eliminates the pain many women experience just before ovulation. It also protects against benign breast disease and reduces the risk of complications associated with ovarian cysts. Lifetime risk of developing ovarian or endometrial cancer is reduced by as much as 40 to 50 percent.

Aren't birth control pills dangerous?

There are innumerable myths surrounding the birth control pill. Let's try to separate fact from fiction.

The most serious complication of oral contraceptives is deep-vein thrombosis. In this condition, a blood clot develops in the deep veins of

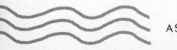

the leg. If a portion of this clot dislodges, it can travel to the lungs. This is a rare event, particularly with modern pills. However, women using oral contraceptives should call the doctor immediately if they develop severe leg pain, chest pain, or shortness of breath. Previously, there have been concerns regarding other cardiovascular problems such as strokes and heart attacks. Recent studies indicate no increased risk of these in nonsmokers using low-dose oral contraceptives. Smokers have an increased risk of various cardiovascular complications, and oral contraceptives are not recommended for smokers over age 35.

Women who are vulnerable to migraine headaches should use oral contraceptives with caution. If headaches become more severe than usual or if eye problems such as blurred or double vision develop, it is safer to choose a different method of contraception.

The greatest concern women have about the birth control pill is cancer. Most studies show that the pill does not increase the risk of cervical cancer. A recent review of studies from around the world suggests that women using oral contraceptives have a slightly higher detection of localized breast cancer (one that hasn't spread beyond the breast). It is difficult to know whether this is a real increase or just reflects earlier diagnosis among women who use birth control pills, because these women are given regular breast exams and are more likely to undergo mammography. The review notes that women on the pill have a lower incidence of advanced breast cancer compared to nonusers. The small increase in breast cancer in women who use birth control pills disappears ten or more years after they stop, suggesting that there is little or no increase in the overall risk. Women who use the pill are far less likely to get endometrial and ovarian cancer. The decrease in ovarian cancer is particularly significant, since this is the most difficult gynecologic cancer to detect, often appearing in its advanced stages before being discovered.

Two other uncommon complications are worth mentioning. Women who are predisposed to high blood pressure may have a greater chance of developing it while using oral contraceptives. Very rarely, oral contraceptives induce the development of a liver tumor. The risk is approximated at 3 women per 100,000 users.

For most women who require reliable contraception, the benefits of

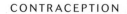

the pill outweigh the risks. There are far greater risks associated with pregnancy.

The birth control pill is not recommended for the following groups:

- Smokers over age 35
- Women who have a history of uterine or breast cancer
- Women who have a history of active liver dysfunction such as hepatitis
- Women who have a history of vascular disease (blood clots, stroke, heart attack)
- Women who have unexplained vaginal bleeding

What about all the side effects from the pill?

Almost every symptom known to humanity has been popularly associated with the pill. In reality, 90 percent of women who try the pill do well with it. Common side effects include nausea, bloating, headaches, mood changes, breast tenderness, and bleeding between periods. Most side effects will decrease after the first few months. If they are particularly severe, the doctor can prescribe a different brand. One common myth is that oral contraceptives induce weight gain. Studies indicate that just as many women lose weight as gain weight on the pill.

It is common to miss a menstrual period on the pill. This is a source of distress for the woman who assumes this means that she is pregnant. Actually her chances of pregnancy are less than 1 percent. In this case, there are no adverse consequences of missing a period. The lining of the uterus simply didn't thicken sufficiently for menstrual flow. If no pills were missed that month, the next pack can be started without concern. If pills were missed, the doctor should be consulted.

Are there any medications I can't take with the pill?

There are no adverse cross-reactions between the pill and other medications. However, some medications may decrease the efficacy of the pill or increase the chances of bleeding between periods. Drugs that have been associated with this include the following:

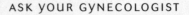

- Rifampin, ampicillin, and tetracycline (antibiotics)
- Barbiturates, Tegretol, and Dilantin (antiseizure medications)
- Phenylbutazone (an anti-inflammatory drug)
- Griseofulvin (an antifungal medication)

If you are taking one of these medications for a short period of time, it is probably safest to use a backup method of contraception such as the condom. That way you don't have to worry. If you will have to be on the medication for a long time, consult your gynecologist.

What should I do if I miss a pill?

It is not uncommon to forget a pill or to drop it down the drain. Don't panic! Take two the next day, or as soon as you remember to. Take them at different times of the day to reduce the likelihood of nausea. Expect spotting when missing a pill. If you miss more than one pill, use a backup method of protection and call your doctor for instructions.

Will I have trouble getting pregnant when I stop taking the pill?

Oral contraceptives do not affect fertility. Infertility is a common problem, affecting one in five couples. However, studies comparing previous pill users and nonusers reveal no difference in pregnancy rates.

What about the minipill?

Is this just a smaller version of the real thing? Well, not quite. The minipill is an oral contraceptive containing only progesterone — the more common birth control pills have both estrogen and progesterone. It is often prescribed for women who should not take estrogen because they are prone to conditions such as blood clots. It is also useful for women who experience estrogen-related side effects when using combination birth control pills. There are two main problems with minipills. First, they are not as effective as combination birth control pills. The failure rate is 1 to 5 percent. Second, erratic bleeding is common. This poses no danger but is rather disconcerting.

What is the "morning after" pill?

The passion of the moment took over, and you had unprotected intercourse. Now what do you do? You may be a candidate for using oral contraceptives in the "morning after" regimen (also called emergency contraception). Two medium-dose birth control pills are taken within 12 to 24 hours after unprotected sex, followed by two more 12 hours later (other variations exist, but this is the most common). The pills alter the inside lining of the uterus, decreasing your chances of becoming pregnant. Although you should start this regimen within the first 24 hours after you have unprotected intercourse, it may be effective up to 72 hours after. Because you are using an increased dose of oral contraceptives, your chances of side effects, particularly nausea, are increased. Your doctor can give you antinausea medicine before you take the birth control pills. This regimen is not foolproof and should be supervised by your doctor. Emergency contraception can also be used if a condom slips off or breaks, or if a diaphragm slips out of place. You can also obtain information by calling an emergency contraception hotline (800-584-9911).

Are IUDs safe?

The IUD, short for intrauterine device, got its bad reputation from the Dalkon Shield, a particular type of IUD that caused a high incidence of pelvic infections. The Dalkon Shield received much publicity, resulting in multiple lawsuits. The adverse publicity resulted in a decline in IUD usage, which is unfortunate, because it is a good choice for many women.

The IUD is a plastic device inserted into the uterus by a doctor. It contains either copper or progesterone. Periodically (annually for progesterone, every ten years for copper) it is removed, and a new IUD is inserted. When conception is desired, it is removed. The IUD is 98 percent successful in preventing pregnancy. Little is required of the woman, so it is convenient.

Sounds great! What's the catch? The IUD increases the risk of developing PID, or pelvic inflammatory disease. Although this risk is small with today's IUDs (approximately 1 to 2 percent), the conse-

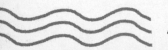

quences can be severe. With every pelvic infection, there is a chance of developing scar tissue, called adhesions, which may in turn result in infertility or chronic pelvic pain. Women in a mutually monogamous relationship who are at low risk for contracting sexually transmitted diseases have minimal risk of developing PID. However, IUDs are not recommended for women who are interested in childbearing, unless they are willing to accept this risk. For a woman who has completed her family but does not want permanent sterilization, the IUD is an excellent choice.

Another drawback of the IUD is the tendency to cause crampier and heavier menstrual periods. Usually this side effect occurs in the first few cycles, but sometimes it persists. As a result, 20 percent of women discontinue use of the IUD.

Although pregnancy rarely occurs if an IUD is in proper position, serious complications can result when it does. There is an increased risk of miscarriage, ectopic pregnancy (also called tubal pregnancy), premature delivery, and uterine infection. If you miss a period while using an IUD, contact your doctor. If pregnancy is confirmed, he or she will recommend removal of the IUD. Although its removal increases your chances of miscarriage, it decreases the risks of serious complications late in the pregnancy.

IUDs provide safe, reliable contraception. Serious complications are uncommon. However, if you experience any of the following, contact your doctor immediately:

- Persistent pain very low in the abdomen

- Persistent fever

- Prolonged bleeding (for more than a week) or a missed period

- Inability to locate the IUD's string, or feeling hard plastic when checking for the string

How can I tell if my IUD is in place?

Every IUD has a string attached to it. The doctor trims the string so that approximately one-half inch to one inch protrudes into the vagina from the cervix. Prior to intercourse, place a finger in the vagina and feel for this string, which feels like fishing line. First, locate your cervix, which feels like the tip of your nose. The string emanates from the opening of the cervix. If you feel a hard plastic piece, it indicates that the uterus has expelled your IUD. Expulsion most commonly occurs within the first few weeks after insertion, but it can happen at any time. Most women generally have no problems with the IUD. But if you can't feel your string, one of three events has happened:

- The uterus has expelled the IUD. It must be replaced.

- The string has simply retracted into the uterus, but the IUD remains in place. An ultrasound scan can confirm this diagnosis, and no further treatment will be needed.

- The IUD has perforated the uterus — a very rare but potentially serious complication. It must be removed. Laparoscopy may be necessary. Contact your doctor if you cannot feel your string.

What is the birth control device that is placed in the arm?

The Norplant system contains rods made of flexible plastic that are placed immediately under the skin in the upper arm. The rods are injected with progesterone that gradually is released into the body. Norplant is very effective at preventing pregnancy and has a failure rate of less than 1 percent. After being inserted under local anesthesia, the rods may be allowed to remain in place for five years. At the end of that time, they are removed under local anesthesia, and new ones can be put in. Because they contain progesterone, they may cause some of the same side effects that occur with use of birth control pills: nausea, headaches, bloating, breast tenderness, and mood changes. However, the majority of women tolerate Norplant well, with few side effects.

Norplant's biggest drawbacks are its high price and the erratic bleeding it can cause. Including the physician's fee for insertion and removal, the cost is $500 to $1,000. Because it contains only progesterone, erratic bleeding is common, particularly in the first year of usage. Although the bleeding is not dangerous and is often controlled by taking estrogen for a short period of time, many women discontinue use of Norplant because of this side effect.

Norplant was introduced into the U.S. market in 1991 after extensive use in other countries. Recently, it has come under attack, and in a number of lawsuits it has been claimed that the product is harmful. Allegations include that Norplant causes weight gain, mood swings, excessive bleeding, and painful removals that result in scars and infection. Yet with the exception of the difficulty experienced by some physicians in removing the implants, most of these side effects can accompany the use of any hormonal contraceptive. As physicians gain experience with insertion and removal, difficult removals become less frequent. Seek an experienced provider if you choose this method.

I hear that there are shots that prevent pregnancy. Is that true?

You heard correctly. A progesterone injection called Depo-Provera can be injected into the arm and will slowly release the hormone into the body. A shot of it every three months provides reliable contraception. Available for decades in this country, this hormonal preparation was not approved for contraceptive use because studies linked it to breast tumors in beagles. Since then, researchers have found that it does not cause tumors in people. Others have raised concerns that women who use Depo-Provera for a long time may suffer loss of bone density. The risk appears to be small, however.

Side effects with Depo-Provera are similar to those of Norplant: nausea, bloating, headaches, breast tenderness, and mood changes. In addition, weight commonly increases by five to ten pounds. The most common reason for discontinuing the use of Depo-Provera is erratic bleeding. Adverse reactions may persist for as long as four months, since the progesterone is slowly released over the course of three months. Its contraceptive effect can persist even after it is discontinued. Therefore, it is not a good choice for those who plan to get pregnant in the near future.

How do I know which method of contraception is best for me?

No single method of contraception is right for everyone. This decision must be made in conjunction with your doctor. Here are a few guidelines:

- If you wish to avoid "artificial" contraception, natural family planning is your only choice. Keep in mind that it is the most difficult and least successful of contraceptive methods.

- If you are single and sexually active, birth control pills are probably your best choice, since they are the most effective at preventing pregnancy. Unless you are involved in a stable, mutually monogamous relationship, condoms should also be used to protect you against sexually transmitted diseases.

- If you are notoriously unreliable in taking oral contraceptives regularly, the IUD and Norplant system are good choices. Once in place, these offer excellent protection and require little or no effort on your part.

- If your goal is to use the safest contraceptives with the fewest side effects, barrier methods (see page 36) are your best choice. However, you must combine multiple barrier methods to approach the effectiveness of hormonal contraceptives. Barrier contraceptives also tend to disrupt foreplay, so you must be highly motivated to use them effectively.

- If you have completed your family, sterilization (tubal ligation or vasectomy) may be the best bet. You should consider this only if permanent contraception is your goal.

How are abortions done?

There are two commonly used practices for electively terminating pregnancy. D&E, or dilation and evacuation, is typically performed if the pregnancy is early (up to 12 to 14 weeks from the last menstrual period). A labor-inducing form of abortion is used when the pregnancy is more advanced.

A D&E, also referred to as suction curettage, is usually performed as an outpatient procedure in either an office setting or surgical facility. The pregnancy is confirmed by a blood pregnancy test or pelvic ultrasound. The doctor administers a local anesthetic in or near the cervix. Sedatives may also be given. If the pregnancy is more advanced, general anesthesia is administered. The doctor dilates the cervix and inserts a plastic tube that is connected to a suction pump. The pregnancy is then

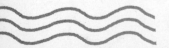

ASK YOUR GYNECOLOGIST

evacuated. After a period of observation (one to three hours), the patient can go home. A variable degree of cramping and bleeding will follow the procedure. Activities may be restricted after the procedure, although most can be resumed within a day or two.

Elective abortion of more advanced pregnancies (14 to 24 weeks from the last menstrual period) is accomplished by using agents that induce labor. They may be administered as a vaginal suppository, parenteral (intravenous or intramuscular) injection, or uterine injection. Labor contractions begin within 12 hours, and the pregnancy is expelled within 12 to 24 hours. If the placenta ("afterbirth") is not expelled spontaneously, a D&E is performed. The most common agents used to induce contractions are prostaglandins, those naturally occurring substances released from the uterus that cause menstrual cramping. Side effects from prostaglandins include nausea, vomiting, diarrhea, and fever. Medications are given before and during the induction to decrease the severity of these side effects. Labor-inducing abortions are usually performed in the hospital and may require an overnight stay.

Some physicians perform an extended D&E on advanced pregnancies. In addition to suction curettage, special instruments are used to evacuate the pregnancy from the uterus. An extended D&E has several advantages over induced labor. The painful contractions of labor are avoided, as are the side effects from the prostaglandins. The procedure is also less time consuming. If the physician is inexperienced, however, there is significant risk of uterine perforation and hemorrhage.

Complications from abortion include bleeding, infection, and uterine perforation. Serious complications are rare. Pain that lasts for more than a day or two, heavy bleeding, fever, or nausea and vomiting should prompt a call to the gynecologist.

Early pregnancy is highly dependent on progesterone, one of the ovarian hormones. RU-486, or mifepristone, is an antiprogestational agent that has been used extensively in Europe to induce abortion early in pregnancy — less than seven to nine weeks from the last menstrual period. Regimens using RU-486 typically involve three outpatient visits. The RU-486 is given at the first visit. Thirty-six to 48 hours later, a prostaglandin is administered. Complete expulsion of the pregnancy is confirmed at a third visit. A D&E is performed if the abortion is incomplete. Side effects include painful uterine contractions, nausea, vomiting, diarrhea, and headache. Use of RU-486 in the United States has been limited, so many physicians will not have experience with this regimen.

The effects abortion may have on your emotional state depend on your values, your circumstances, and your religious beliefs. Depending on your circumstances, consultation with a health care professional, counselor, psychologist, social worker, or religious leader may be beneficial.

Can I have a normal pregnancy after having an abortion?

Most physicians agree that an uncomplicated abortion will have no impact on subsequent pregnancies. There is always a small chance that a severe complication could have an effect on your future fertility, but this is uncommon. Fewer studies have looked at the effect of multiple abortions on fertility. Multiple abortions may increase the risk of preterm birth in later pregnancies.

How is a tubal ligation done? Is it safe?

A common question is "How do they tie your tubes?" Actually, the term is a misnomer because tubes are not usually tied. Except for sterilization performed immediately after delivery, tubal ligations are done as outpatient surgery, utilizing laparoscopy. After administering anesthesia, the doctor expands the abdominal cavity by filling it with gas. A telescopic instrument is inserted through a tiny incision near the navel to permit a view of the pelvic organs. A section of one fallopian tube is grasped and is coagulated (an electric current is passed through the tube), clipped, or banded. The doctor performs a similar procedure on the other tube. Depending on the technique used, a second small incision may be necessary. The incisions (less than one-half inch in length) are easily closed. After a period of observation in a recovery area, the patient is discharged and may resume normal activities the following day.

Occasionally, the procedure cannot be completed through the laparoscope, and a larger incision is required to finish the operation, which might lengthen hospitalization and recovery. If this is unacceptable, let your doctor know in advance.

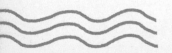

Recovery from laparoscopic sterilization is usually uneventful. It is common to experience discomfort in the shoulder for a day or two. The cause is actually residual gas in the abdominal cavity, but the brain mistakenly attributes it to the shoulder. The body will absorb the gas, and the symptom will disappear. If you experience nausea from the anesthesia or surgery, eat lightly until it clears, usually within 24 hours. Pain may be felt in the pelvic region or at abdominal incisions. Your doctor can give you prescriptions to relieve pain and nausea before you leave the hospital.

Complications with laparoscopic tubal sterilization are uncommon. They include bleeding and injury to other internal organs such as the bowel, ureters, and bladder, and their repair may require a more extensive operation. The possibility of complications should not deter a woman from choosing this operation, however, because they are rare.

The failure rate for tubal sterilization is less than 1 percent. When pregnancy does occur, there is a greater than normal chance that it will be a tubal one. Tubal pregnancies are life threatening if not detected early. If you miss a period after undergoing tubal sterilization, contact your doctor.

Can my tubes be put back together?

A tubal ligation should not be considered reversible. If there is any chance that you might want to become pregnant in the future, tubal sterilization should not be performed. Having said that, we realize life doesn't always lead down the expected paths. The loss of a child or a second marriage often motivates women to try to get their tubal ligations reversed.

To rejoin the severed tubes, infertility specialists perform tubal reanastomosis. For this operation to be successful, a large proportion of the tubes must be healthy. If there is sufficient tubal length to allow the procedure, success rates are 50 percent. If the tubes are beyond salvage, you should consider in vitro fertilization. In this procedure, your eggs are retrieved from the ovary, fertilized outside the body, and then introduced into the uterus, bypassing the tubes.

Why have my periods been irregular since my tubes were tied?

Although it often seems that there is a change in one's menses in the years following a tubal ligation, most investigators who have looked into this question have not found a greater incidence of menstrual abnormalities among women who have undergone that operation. One reason for the apparent rise in problems following tubal ligations is that most women undergo tubal ligation in their middle to late thirties, a time when periods normally start to exhibit more variation.

Is it better for my husband to have a vasectomy than for me to undergo a tubal ligation?

It certainly is easier. Most of the male reproductive tract is outside the body, making it more accessible. Sperm is made in the testes and then transported through tubes called the vas deferens. Under local anesthesia, they can be easily cut and sealed, thereby preventing the release of sperm from the testes. Minor swelling and discomfort are typical, but serious complications or side effects are rare.

The main drawback of vasectomy is that, unlike tubal ligation, it is not immediately effective. A backup method of contraception must be used until the doctor determines that no sperm are present on semen analysis. This may take as long as several months.

Men often avoid vasectomy because of the misimpression that it will interfere with sexual performance or enjoyment. Vasectomy does not interfere with arousal, erection, or ejaculation.

Vasectomy is very reliable, with a failure rate of less than 1 percent. Although putting the tubes back together may be successful, you should not consider vasectomy reversible.

If I'm in menopause, can I still get pregnant?

First, make sure you're really in menopause. You may think you are menopausal if you are over 40 and not having menstrual periods. However, it is possible that your cycle is "out of sync" but your ovaries are still active. If this is the case, you might still ovulate and conceive. If you

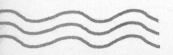

are not having menstrual periods and are experiencing hot flashes, it is probable that you are menopausal. This can be confirmed through measuring hormone levels through bloodwork. Once menopause is confirmed, continue to use a method of contraception for at least another 6 to 12 months. Occasionally, a woman will still manage to ovulate within this time — a kind of "last hurrah."

 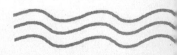

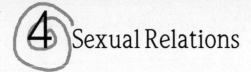

4 Sexual Relations

Why does it hurt when I have sex?

It doesn't seem fair. Your reproductive organs cause you grief your whole life. Your menstrual period disrupts your life at the most inopportune times. On top of that, cramps accompany it. There is a litany of things that can go wrong with the reproductive organs. At the very least, you deserve to get some pleasure from them. Isn't that where sex enters the picture? You hope so. Therefore, it is particularly distressing when you experience pain during sexual encounters. What should be intimate and pleasurable is transformed into a frightening, painful experience. This extends beyond the physical pain to affect your emotional well-being. If the problem is recurrent, it may also strain a relationship.

If intercourse is painful, seek help. You must overcome any embarrassment you may have about discussing this with your doctor. Trust us: Your problem is not unique, and the doctor can't help you if you don't ask.

There are numerous causes for painful intercourse. We'll start our discussion with the most common causes and gradually work our way toward those that are more obscure.

The most likely cause for discomfort in the vagina during intercourse is insufficient lubrication. Vaginal lubrication naturally happens as sexual arousal occurs; the vagina moistens with secretions produced by the vaginal walls. Without adequate foreplay, lubrication will not occur. Some men think getting undressed constitutes ample foreplay, so you might have to give your partner a clue as to what is required for you to become stimulated. Sexual arousal is more difficult when you are anxious, so try to initiate sex in a relaxed setting.

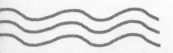

Vaginal dryness is normal at some points in life. The weeks immediately following childbirth are one such time. If you breast-feed your infant, dryness will continue longer. As your estrogen production resumes, the problem will correct itself. You will also develop vaginal dryness at menopause. Estrogen replacement will help, if you choose to pursue hormonal replacement therapy (see chapter 13). Vaginal moisturizing creams (Replens and Gyne-moistren) can be purchased over the counter for generalized vaginal dryness. However, if your problem is painful intercourse, you should use a lubricant. Lubricants can be purchased without a prescription in the form of a cream, jelly, or suppository. The cheapest is ordinary K-Y jelly, which gynecologists often use for examinations. All lubricants are water-based preparations that do not stain and clean up readily. Do not use a petroleum- or oil-based product such as Vaseline, particularly if your partner uses latex condoms, because the petroleum jelly dissolves latex.

Vaginitis, inflammation of the vagina, is another common cause of painful intercourse. Suspect an infection if you have vaginal burning or itching. An unusual discharge or odor may also be present. Although the infection may begin in the vagina, it can spread externally to create inflammation of the vulva (called vulvitis). Examples include yeast infections, trichomoniasis, and bacterial vaginosis. Other infections cause ulceration of the vulva or opening of the vagina. Herpes and syphilis can both do this. Of the two, herpes is more likely to cause painful open sores that prevent intercourse. Genital warts (condylomata) commonly affect the external genitalia and can produce pain. We will discuss these infections in more detail in chapter 5.

Vulvar inflammation and sensitivity (see chapter 11) can also arise from an irritant or allergic reaction. A few suggestions are worth emphasizing. Use only mild soaps without deodorants, scents, and dyes (a good choice is white, unscented Dove). Use white, unscented toilet paper. Wear white cotton underclothing, and wash your underclothing with mild detergents.

Various dermatologic diseases produce vulvar inflammation, making intercourse painful. The doctor diagnoses these either by their appearance or after a skin biopsy, which can be done in the office under local anesthesia. Your gynecologist or dermatologist can treat these with anti-inflammatory creams or ointments to reduce the inflammation.

Vaginismus, painful spasm of the vagina that precludes intercourse, may also cause pain on attempted entry. Muscles at the opening of the vagina often tighten in anticipation of pain. If you have experienced painful attempts at intercourse previously, or have been sexually abused, this is more likely to happen.

The good news is that you can learn to control these muscles. Place one finger into the vagina, and attempt to contract the muscles around your finger. Now concentrate on relaxing the muscles. Continue to do this until you achieve control. Once you have established control, introduce a second finger and repeat the sequence. Finally, overlap three fingers (place your second and fourth fingers under your third finger). When you can successfully introduce three overlapped fingers and still relax your muscles, intercourse should be possible. It is important not to attempt intercourse prior to this point. If you try too soon, you will feel pain, which makes it more difficult to learn vaginal muscle relaxation.

Some women prefer to use vaginal dilators for their relaxation exercises. They are available in sets of four graduated sizes. Before attempting intercourse, concentrate on sexual foreplay to help with vaginal lubrication and relaxation. Digital stimulation, with your partner placing his fingers in your vagina, is helpful. See if you can relax your vaginal muscles while your partner puts his fingers in. You can then attempt intercourse. Don't hesitate to use a lubricant (K-Y jelly is fine), and lower yourself from above onto his penis. That way you have control over the degree of penetration. You can lower yourself slowly, stopping intermittently to relax the vaginal muscles.

Sometimes, the opening of the vagina is partly closed by the hymen, a ring of tissue located at the entrance to the vagina. Your doctor can assess this and instruct you on how to stretch the hymenal ring, using your fingers or vaginal dilators. If this is unsuccessful, the doctor can make small incisions (while you are under anesthesia) to open the hymenal ring.

A cyst or abscess in the special glands located between the labia, at the entrance to the vaginal canal in what is called the vestibule, can

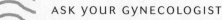

cause pain with attempted entry into the vagina. They can be treated with warm compresses, incision and drainage, or removal. A local or generalized inflammation limited to the vestibule, known as vulvar vestibulitis, can also be the problem. The inflammation is often overlooked on examination but causes intense pain when touched. Vestibular disorders are discussed more thoroughly in chapter 11.

Urinary tract infections occasionally cause painful intercourse, but not usually. The bladder and urethra lie in direct proximity to the vagina. The opening of the urethra, called the urethral meatus, is located immediately above the vaginal opening. Inflammation associated with cystitis (bladder infection) or urethritis (urethral infection) may cause pain either with initial penetration of the vagina or during intercourse. Other common symptoms of urinary infections include frequency (you feel as if you have to run to the bathroom every five minutes), urgency (you feel as though you'd better get there quickly or have an accident), and pain or burning when you urinate.

Pain that occurs with deep penetration is the most serious problem, as it may represent a disorder of the internal reproductive organs. Uterine infections (not to be confused with vaginal infections) may cause pain with deep penetration. Treatment consists of antibiotics. Other uterine problems such as fibroids (noncancerous tumors in the wall of the uterus) and adenomyosis (a condition in which the inside lining of the uterus grows into the wall of the uterus) may create pain when the penis hits the cervix. Ovaries are very sensitive, and cysts or tumors of the ovaries increase the likelihood of experiencing pain with deep penetration. Endometriosis and pelvic adhesions also create pain felt deep in the pelvis. A thorough examination and pelvic ultrasound are warranted when there is deep pelvic pain during intercourse. If the results of the tests are normal, you should try different positions. You may have less pain if you control the degree of penetration by positioning yourself on top during intercourse. If the problem is persistent and severe, you should consider laparoscopy (see page 21).

Rarely, pain in the vagina results from scarring related to previous vaginal surgery or injuries incurred during childbirth. These areas may stretch and become less painful with time. Anesthetic creams or lubricants may help. Experiment with different positions during intercourse.

If the vagina is narrowed, vaginal dilators can be used to increase the width of the vagina. Surgery is indicated if no improvement is seen over time. There is always a small chance that the operation will produce scarring that might worsen the condition. Therefore, it is best to pursue conservative options before proceeding with surgery.

Finally, emotional factors can influence sexual response. Problems within a relationship, depression, anxiety, and emotional or sexual abuse all interfere with the natural sexual response, inhibiting relaxation of the muscles at the opening of the vagina and decreasing vaginal lubrication. The lengthening of the vagina that occurs with a normal sexual response may be inhibited, allowing the penis to hit sensitive structures deep within the pelvis. All of these can produce pain, which causes more emotional distress, further restricting the natural sexual response. A vicious cycle develops, which becomes progressively harder to break. Depression or anxiety that interferes with your sex life warrants evaluation by a psychologist or psychiatrist. A strained relationship may benefit from marriage counseling. Deal with the problem, and seek help early before it becomes overwhelming.

Why don't I have orgasms?

We're presuming that you see this as a problem. Lack of an orgasm is a problem only if you or your partner perceive it as one. Having said that, approximately 90 percent of women can experience orgasm. The inability to achieve one frequently relates to misconceptions about the normal sexual response. This response consists of four phases:

Excitement Phase The sexual response begins with sexual arousal. With excitement, the clitoris enlarges and hardens. The clitoris is a swelling located immediately above the vaginal and urethral openings. There is a "hood," or fold of tissue, overlying it that often retracts during this phase, making the clitoris more accessible. The clitoris is far more sensitive than any other structure in the genital region and is almost always responsible for initiating orgasm. Difficulty achieving orgasm is most typically the result of insufficient stimulation of the clitoris. Women generally require prolonged stimulation of this and other erogenous areas in order to experience orgasm. Occasionally, the

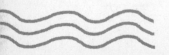

clitoris is so sensitive that direct stimulation is painful. This can be overcome by stimulation of the tissues adjacent to the clitoris, while avoiding direct contact.

Explore your body to identify other areas that arouse you. Pleasurable places may include the breasts (particularly the nipples), ears, neck, vagina, buttocks, anus, thighs, and feet. You must communicate with your partner and direct him to the areas that provide pleasurable sensations for you. This is no time to be shy. Assertiveness in the bedroom has its distinct rewards (although assertiveness is best exerted gradually . . . you don't want to scare the poor guy). Men often become excited and experience orgasm quickly. He needs to understand that this is not a race. Tell him that he needs to be more attentive for an extended time before and after intercourse. Try to have sex in a relaxed setting when neither of you are pressed for time. Leave your stress and tension at the bedroom door. Try to let your mind focus on the pleasurable sensations that you are experiencing, not on whether Billy did his homework and Susie finished her piano practice.

During the excitement phase, the vagina moistens with secretions. Blood begins to engorge the internal and external genitalia, which may be noticed by swelling of the labia. The vagina begins to lengthen and expand to readily accept the penis. The uterus swells and rises from its usual position. The nipples may become erect and more sensitive to stimulation.

Plateau Phase During this phase excitement continues to build. The pelvic structures become further engorged. The vagina continues to expand. At this point the clitoris retracts under its hood. If sexual response stops at this phase without progression to orgasm, "pelvic congestion syndrome" may occur. In this disorder, the pelvic region remains engorged with blood, resulting in pelvic soreness or aching and sometimes backache. It can be relieved by continuing stimulation until orgasm is reached.

Orgasm Phase The peak of the cycle brings extremely pleasurable sensations in association with rhythmic contractions of the vagina and uterus. The anal muscles tighten, and the toes may curl. After a short period of time this abates, and muscular tension relaxes.

Resolution Phase Following the orgasm, a woman may return to the plateau phase. If stimulated at this time, she may again achieve orgasm. Some women will experience multiple orgasms during sex. If there is no further stimulation, the pelvic organs and genitalia return to their prearoused state.

There is tremendous variability in sexual responsiveness. Orgasms may be experienced at varying levels of intensity, and not all sexual encounters will culminate in orgasm. Sexual intimacy should be about love and sharing, not performance. Focusing on performance produces tension and anxiety that decreases the chance of having a fulfilling sensual experience.

If you can't allow yourself to relax and enjoy the pleasurable sensations provided through sexual stimulation, your chances of reaching orgasm are diminished. Your inhibitions may result from a misconception that sex is "dirty." This is often the message that parents inadvertently (or not so inadvertently) transmit to their children. Some mothers have told their daughters that sex is a duty, performed for the man's enjoyment and not the woman's. This misimpression doesn't change overnight. However, with a supportive partner you should be able to gradually allow yourself to experience the pleasure you deserve. If you still have difficulty, consider sexual counseling.

Drugs, alcohol, and certain medications may decrease your ability to become sexually aroused and reach orgasm. Alcohol may initially lower your inhibitions and therefore increase your ability to enjoy sex. However, it depresses the central nervous system and ultimately decreases response to sexual stimulation. Some medications decrease libido (sexual desire) or sexual responsiveness. Check with your physician if you are taking medications and have this problem. The *Physician's Desk Reference* will state whether decreased libido is a side effect.

Certain medical disorders, such as depression or anxiety, may interfere with your sexual responsiveness, as do chronic medical illnesses. Lowered hormone levels experienced by nursing mothers may decrease sexual arousal, and chronic fatigue and sleep deprivation may play their part as well: "I don't see him getting up to nurse the baby." Lowered hormone levels during menopause may decrease libido. Hormonal replacement, particularly if testosterone is included, can help (see page 167).

Where is the "G spot"?

OK, you got us. This is not a frequently asked question, but it was too good to pass up. One can't talk about orgasm without at least mentioning the famous "G spot," or Grafenberg spot. This is a swelling in the upper front section of your vaginal wall that is reputed to create orgasmic arousal. Stimulation of this area is thought to elicit a "vaginal orgasm." Some physicians do not acknowledge the existence of the G spot. They feel that vaginal stimulation indirectly transmits neural impulses through the clitoris to induce sexual excitement. Finding the G spot is certainly not critical for a fulfilling sexual experience. Nevertheless, think of all the fun you will have trying to locate it.

Why don't I have any sex drive?

The loss of sex drive is extremely disconcerting. Many times the decrease in libido is related to factors in your life. With the frantic pace of couples' lives today, it is difficult to find time to relax and reach the degree of intimacy necessary for romance. Work may leave either partner "stressed out" or exhausted. It's unrealistic to expect a sex drive to thrive under those circumstances.

It is important that you make time for you and your partner to be alone. A vacation away from work with just the two of you is ideal. It gives you the opportunity to forget all the complications of your life and to focus on each other. If that much time away is not possible, aim for a weekend or even just a day. Devote more time to thoughts and activities that enhance sex. Men usually spend more of each day thinking about sex than women do. It's no wonder they are often raring to go. Discover (or rediscover) activities that sexually arouse you. Sometimes reading romantic or erotic novels or magazines will intensify your sexual drive. Sexual fantasy may also heighten your desire for an encounter. It is unrealistic to spend your entire day without sexual thoughts and then to expect to instantly turn on your libido when needed.

Fear is a great libido killer. If you're afraid of getting pregnant, consult your doctor for a contraceptive that ensures adequate protection. A fear of being hurt may stem from misconceptions regarding sex. Educate yourself regarding sexual techniques, and advise your partner of your concerns so that he will be more sensitive to your problem. If you have experienced pain during sexual encounters, see your gynecologist prior to attempting intercourse again (see page 52). Tell your partner about any psychological fears, such as a fear of losing control or of being emotionally hurt. Consultation with a therapist may be useful.

Illnesses that sap your strength will also zap your sex drive. But if you have unlimited stamina yet simply no interest in sex, it is unlikely a physical disorder is causing the problem. However, if fatigue extends to the other areas of your life, a good physical exam and possibly some lab work should be scheduled. Depression is associated with decreased libido and must be treated if sexual desire is to resume. Some medications decrease libido as a side effect. If the problem appears to coincide with starting a particular medication, check with your doctor. Perhaps substitutes are available.

Probably the least common cause for decreased libido is a hormonal disturbance. The female hormones, particularly estrogen, may influence sex drive. However, most of the sex drive derives from androgens. You may be thinking, "Wait a minute, aren't androgens male hormones?" They are indeed. But women also produce androgens from their ovaries and adrenal glands. It is uncommon for women with functioning ovaries to have decreased androgen levels, but they may occur in women who use oral contraceptives. This problem may be overcome by changing to a different formulation. The decrease in estrogen and androgens during menopause may also lower libido. If estrogen replacement does not solve the problem, you should consider adding a small amount of testosterone to your hormonal regimen (see page 167).

Will my sexual pleasure decrease after a hysterectomy?

After hysterectomy, uterine contractions will no longer occur during orgasm. Very occasionally, some women may experience a decrease in enjoyment from this change. Most sexual arousal, however, is generated through either direct or indirect stimulation of the clitoris and is not altered by hysterectomy. A slight shortening of the vagina results from hysterectomy but is inconsequential to successful intercourse. A hysterectomy without removal of the ovaries does not alter hormone production. If the ovaries are removed at the time of hysterectomy and hormone replacement is not begun, vaginal dryness and problems with libido can arise. Occasionally, postoperative adhesions (scars) at the top of the vagina will cause painful intercourse during deep penetration. This condition is uncommon and can often be overcome by changing position during intercourse or limiting the degree of penetration. In severe cases, surgery may be required to release the adhesions.

Psychological factors can play a positive or negative role in your sex life after hysterectomy. It has been our experience that hysterectomy often has a positive psychological impact. Often much distress has been associated with the uterine disorder. You may have had a long-standing history of prolonged or erratic bleeding. Your condition may have caused chronic or recurring pelvic pain. A multitude of treatments may have been attempted without success. After hysterectomy, life can return to normal and your interest in sex can return. Strained interpersonal relationships also improve with resolution of your long-standing ailment. If a fear of pregnancy has been restricting your ability to relax and enjoy sex, you may find greater sexual freedom after the hysterectomy.

For some women, however, losing the capacity for childbearing may be difficult to accept. If this is the case, hysterectomy can have a profound emotional impact that diminishes sexual responsiveness. You may be able to overcome this problem on your own, but don't hesitate to consult a therapist if you cannot resolve these feelings. It is important to discuss these feelings with your partner. His support, along with the reassurance that he still finds you desirable, may help.

In our experience, hysterectomy usually does *not* have a significant impact on sexuality. If your sex life was excellent before the hysterectomy, it will probably remain so after. If it was lousy before, it's not likely to improve because of the surgery. Don't let worries about sex become overriding if a hysterectomy is necessary.

Is oral sex dangerous?

Some sexually transmitted diseases, such as gonorrhea, syphilis, herpes, and yeast infections, can be transmitted through oral sex. Considering the high prevalence of sexually transmitted diseases, however, oral infections are uncommon.

As a rule, if either you or your partner notices an unusual lesion (a wart, ulceration, or skin change) or a discharge, sexual contact of any sort should be put on hold until you find out what's wrong. If a sexually transmittable infection is diagnosed, ask your doctor about any restrictions that may apply regarding sexual activity. Do you need to refrain from all sexual practices while undergoing treatment? Does your partner need to be examined? Will there be any restrictions after treatment? How soon after treatment can you resume normal sexual practices?

Assuming that both of you maintain proper hygiene, there is no danger to you or your partner from oral-genital sex. The mouth and the vagina are both laden with bacteria, but not of the types detrimental to health. There is no harm in ingesting either vaginal secretions or semen.

For additional information regarding sex education or sexual dysfunction, consider contacting the following agencies:

American Association of Sex Educators, Counselors,
    and Therapists
P.O. Box 238
Mount Vernon, IA 52314-0238
(319) 895-8407
www.aasect.org

Council for Sex Information and Education
2272 Colorado Boulevard
No. 1228
Los Angeles, CA 90041

5 Pelvic Infections: Why Do I Itch Down There?

Why do I itch down there?

We'll assume that by "down there," you mean the region of the external genitalia, which are illustrated on page 11. This region includes the following structures:

- *Major (outer) and minor (inner) labia of the vulva:* the lips just outside the vagina
- *Vestibule:* the area between the labia minora at the opening of the vagina
- *Perineum:* the area between the vagina and the anus
- *Clitoris:* the raised area covered by a fold of tissue (called a hood) that is responsible for sexual arousal, located at the top of the labia minora
- *Perianal region:* skin around the anus
- *Urethral meatus:* the opening of the urethra, the tube that empties the bladder, located just above the opening of the vagina

Vaginal and vulvar infections commonly cause itching or burning. Infections that are commonly associated with this include yeast, trichomoniasis, bacterial vaginosis, genital warts, and herpes infections. We'll discuss these one by one.

First, however, you should know that irritant and allergic reactions account for many cases of external itching. If the doctor cannot identify an infectious source for the problem, it is typically caused by one of the following common irritants and allergens:

PELVIC INFECTIONS

- *Soaps that have deodorants, dyes, or scents:* Your best bet is to stick with a mild soap such as Neutrogena or white, unscented Dove.

- *Toilet paper with dyes or scents:* Forget that fancy stuff. Use white, unscented toilet paper.

- *Powders, talcs, and feminine hygiene sprays:* Don't buy into those mother-daughter feminine hygiene moments on TV. You're more likely to create problems than to solve them with those products.

- *Clothing detergents and fabric softeners:* All of that neat stuff they put into detergents to whiten, brighten, and dissolve stains can be quite irritating to your genitalia. Wash your underwear in mild detergents, and rinse them well after washing.

- *Contraceptive products:* Spermicides, condoms, and diaphragms may cause irritation. Chapter 3 presents alternatives to consider if you have this problem.

- *Deodorant pads and tampons:* Again, unscented products are preferable.

Irritant reactions occur immediately upon contact with the offending substance. Allergic reactions may be immediate but usually become more evident hours or days later. Redness and swelling or a rash may be present. If no warts or ulcerations are detected on examination and no infection is identified, an irritant or allergic reaction (also called contact dermatitis) is assumed to be the cause of your discomfort. Your doctor can give you an anti-inflammatory cream (hydrocortisone or something stronger) to resolve the inflammation.

The problem will persist if the offending substance is not eliminated. Wear only white cotton underwear, and if you wear pantyhose, make sure they have a white, cotton inset. Cotton "breathes," whereas synthetic fabrics trap moisture that increases your chance of experiencing irritation and infection. Avoid tight pants for the same reason.

Over-the-counter products that treat "minor vaginal irritation" usually have hydrocortisone or benzocaine as the active ingredient. Avoid the temptation to use these. Serious conditions may be overlooked if you are not examined.

A chronic skin condition, referred to as vulvar dystrophy, can cause burning or itching in the vulvar region. Skin changes may include thinning or thickening, as well as color changes; the skin is usually whiter than normal. In more advanced stages, the opening of the vagina may narrow, and skin ulceration may develop. Your doctor will prescribe a cream or ointment to decrease the itching and prevent worsening of the condition. Treatment must be long-term, and periodic visits are necessary (every three to six months) to monitor the condition. In severe cases in which ulceration has developed, surgery may be required to remove the abnormal skin. Chronic skin conditions that affect other areas of the body, such as psoriasis, may also involve the vulvar region. These skin diseases are usually treated by a dermatologist (a doctor that specializes in skin disorders).

Vulvar cancer may also cause itching (see page 151).

Why do I keep getting yeast infections?

In asking this question, you probably think that you're the only person in the world getting recurrent yeast infections. Actually, yeast infections are quite common, and it is not unusual for women to get them again and again. Yeast and fungi live all around us. They exist in our environment and in our food and are not acquired only through sexual activity. Where does yeast prefer to live? Ideally, it prefers a moist, dark environment. The vagina certainly fits that description.

If you think you have a yeast infection (also referred to as candida vaginitis or monilial vaginitis), your best bet is to see the gynecologist. Commercials for antifungal creams have misled women into thinking that vaginal burning, itching, and discharge always come from yeast infections. However, your symptoms may not be related to yeast. Other types of vaginal infections and other disorders can create similar symptoms. (We discuss infections in this chapter; other vaginal and vulvar conditions are addressed in chapter 11.) If you or your doctor treats your infection without pursuing appropriate diagnostic techniques, you may be treating the wrong problem. All the antifungal medication known to modern medicine won't help if the problem doesn't stem from a fungus. Treating without appropriate diagnosis also makes it more difficult to accurately assess your condition later, should your symptoms persist. Avoid the temptation to treat yourself or to let your doctor treat you by phone, especially if the problem is recurrent. But if your symptoms are severe and it is not practical for the doctor to see you, you might need to make an exception to this rule. A phone consultation is preferable to leaving the matter unresolved. If you do not see any genital lesions (particularly ulcerations or tiny blisters) when you examine yourself by using a hand mirror, it is reasonable for the doctor to prescribe an antifungal medication. If there is severe external burning, the doctor can also prescribe an anti-inflammatory cream (such as hydrocortisone) for immediate relief. However, you should still schedule an appointment to follow up on your treatment.

Once it is determined that your repeated infections are caused by yeast, we're back to your initial question: Why? Use of antibiotics often induces yeast infections in women. It can decrease the normal bacteria in the vagina, allowing the yeast to become dominant. Some women notice a pattern of developing vaginal yeast infections every time they take antibiotics. If this is true for you, it is reasonable to use an antifungal medication following the antibiotics. If you need to be on antibiotics continually, you may need to take an antifungal medication regularly, once or twice per week.

A small percentage of women have yeast infections related to diabetes. Diabetes elevates the sugar level in vaginal secretions, thereby providing an increased food source for the yeast.

The immune system helps fight fungal infections. When this system is compromised, yeast infections persist, recur, or spread to other areas of the body. Drugs that can compromise the immune response include those used in chemotherapy and high doses of cortisone-like steroids. Diseases that compromise the immune defenses, such as leukemia and AIDS, can also set the stage for chronic or repeated yeast infections. If you or your physician has reason to suspect the presence of these diseases, appropriate tests should be ordered. However, remember that these conditions are very uncommon, whereas recurrent yeast infections are very common. Most people with repeated yeast infections do not have a serious underlying illness.

Physicians have debated over the years whether taking oral contraceptives increases the chance of developing vaginal yeast infections. At this point, most doctors do not feel that oral contraceptives significantly increase this risk. If you are having difficulty with yeast infections and are using oral contraceptives, consider stopping them for several months — but only if you can reliably use an alternative method of contraception. If the yeast infections disappear, consider discontinuing oral contraceptives and permanently using a different method.

Most of the time, no reason can be found to explain recurrent yeast infections. However, following these general rules will decrease the likelihood of contracting vaginal infections: Keeping the genital area dry is of paramount importance. You should wear only loose-fitting clothing and cotton undergarments. Synthetic fabrics don't "breathe," and tight clothes trap moisture (remember, yeast likes moisture). If you wear pantyhose, choose a style with a cotton inset. After you shower or bathe, use a blow dryer to ensure that the genital region is dry. Try not to sit around in a wet bathing suit or workout clothes for a prolonged time. After you swim or work out, use the blow dryer and change into dry clothes. Avoid foods containing sugar and sweetened drinks (yeasts loves sugar too).

Are yeast infections dangerous?

Your vaginal yeast infection poses no danger to you. The infection doesn't involve the uterus, fallopian tubes, or ovaries. There is no adverse impact on fertility or childbearing. Vaginal yeast infections do not cause pelvic adhesions or chronic pelvic pain.

Some books propose yeast as a cause for every disorder known to humanity. We have our doubts. Infections spread through the bloodstream are rare, usually affecting only those with a weakened immune system. In a few rare situations, a woman develops an allergic response to yeast. But in general, you can conclude that your yeast infections cause no harm.

How are yeast infections treated?

There are numerous medications designed to treat vaginal yeast infections. Many of these (Monistat, Gyne-Lotrimin, Vagistat, Femstat) are available over the counter. All of them work at least 80 to 90 percent of the time. If you have seen your doctor and yeast infection is diagnosed, it is fine to use one of these products. Vagistat is a particularly good choice since it requires only a single dose and kills many types of fungi. Other antifungal preparations are obtained by prescription. Examples include Terazol (available as a cream or suppository) and Diflucan (a single-dose pill). Avoid the temptation to treat yourself without consulting your gynecologist. If your partner seems fine and has no genital rash or itching, he doesn't need treatment.

Antifungal medications come in a variety of forms. There are creams, suppositories, and tablets. Length of treatment varies from one to seven days. Every physician has a preference, although the method of administration doesn't seem to substantially affect the success rate. It makes sense to use a cream to treat external itching or burning. It should be used externally, as well as in the vagina. Diflucan is the only approved oral medication for vaginal yeast infections. It is taken as a one-dose tablet, certainly the most convenient of the regimens. Its main downside is a 15 percent incidence of headache or gastrointestinal distress, usually minor, for women who take it. Diflucan interacts adversely with certain medications. If you take other medications, check with your physician before starting Diflucan.

Treating recurrent yeast infections can be exasperating. Some physicians will perform fungal cultures to identify the strain of fungus. Sometimes multiple areas will be cultured (mouth, rectum, vagina) to find a possible source for the recurrent infections. However, the testing can get quite expensive. Most physicians take a more pragmatic approach. If you have not used one of the newer antifungal medications, then trying one should be the first step. If your partner has a rash or itch, he should be examined and treated also. If your infection persists or recurs after using one of the newer preparations, you may require a longer course of therapy (two to four weeks). If that fails, try an oral antifungal preparation for an extended period — up to 30 days. The two common medications used for this are Diflucan and Nizoral. Another regimen with proven success is boric acid douches or suppositories used twice daily for two weeks.

Finally, some women's yeast infections will recur no matter what medication or regimen is used. If you fall into this category, you might take an antifungal medication once or twice weekly for several months or longer and then discontinue it, to see if you remain free of infection.

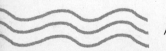

ASK YOUR GYNECOLOGIST

To obtain a free booklet called "A Women's Guide to Vaginal Infections," write to the National Vaginitis Foundation, 117 S. Cook Street, Suite 315, Barrington, IL 60010 (www.vaginalinfections.org).

Will yogurt keep me from getting yeast infections?

No, or at least it is not likely. The idea that yogurt (taken either orally or vaginally) can prevent vaginal infections derives from the presence of lactobacillus in the yogurt. Lactobacillus acidophilus is normally the predominant bacterium of the vagina. When the population of lactobacilli decreases, other organisms such as yeast have an opportunity to overpopulate the vagina. However, a certain strain of lactobacillus is necessary to restore a healthy balance of bacteria in the vagina. Strains that produce hydrogen peroxide must be present. Very few brands of yogurt contain peroxide-producing lactobacillus acidophilus. Others contain lactobacillus acidophilus but are contaminated with unwanted bacteria. Some "natural" health preparations also claim to provide these bacteria (usually referred to as acidophilus on the label). However, these also do not contain a peroxide-producing lactobacillus. Reputable researchers are working to develop preparations that provide these lactobacilli, but no such product is currently available.

I have a discharge but no itching or burning. Is that normal?

It is normal to have a vaginal discharge. The vagina and cervix produce secretions. These secretions, along with vaginal bacteria and exfoliated vaginal cells (surface cells of the vagina that have been shed into the vagina), create a normal discharge. The normal vaginal discharge is clear or white. It should not be particularly "clumpy" or exceedingly "runny," and it should not have an unpleasant odor. It's normal for the discharge to increase in the middle of your menstrual cycle.

If you notice an increase in the amount of discharge, a foul odor, or a change in the color of the discharge, make an appointment to have it evaluated. This secretion may signal a vaginal infection that should be treated. Yeast infections produce a secretion similar to cottage cheese in texture. Usually it is white and does not have a foul odor.

Two other vaginal infections frequently cause an increased discharge. Both usually present a profuse, foul-smelling discharge, but they may

PELVIC INFECTIONS

not be associated with burning or itching. Your only clue may be the increased discharge or odor. The most common of these is bacterial vaginosis, which is actually more common than yeast infections. Most of the time it presents no significant signs of inflammation. The most common symptom is an increased discharge with a foul, "fishy" odor. The condition is caused by a decrease in the number of lactobacilli (the usual dominant bacteria of the vagina), allowing an increase in the population of other bacteria that are normally absent or present in small numbers. One of these is called *Gardnerella*. *Gardnerella* is only one of a number of bacteria that overpopulate the vagina in this condition. The foul odor is caused by substances called amines, which are released by the bacteria. The doctor can easily diagnose the condition by looking at vaginal secretions through a microscope. This test is referred to as a "wet prep."

The doctor will prescribe an antibiotic that selectively decreases the bacteria that have overpopulated the vagina. This gives our friend lactobacillus the chance to reassume its dominant position. The two antibiotics usually used for this are metronidazole (Flagyl) and clindamycin (Cleocin), both of which are available in oral and vaginal preparations. The vaginal preparations are less likely to have side effects but are messier and more expensive. You cannot drink any alcohol during a course of treatment with Flagyl. This is important! You will (we repeat *WILL*) get sick with nausea and vomiting if you combine alcohol with Flagyl. There does not seem to be a higher success rate if your partner is also treated, and most doctors won't do so unless you seem to have frequent recurrences.

The other vaginal infection commonly associated with a profuse, foul discharge is trichomoniasis. It is caused by an organism called *Trichomonas*, which produces a green-yellow discharge, itching or burning, and a foul odor. It, too, is easily diagnosed by a physician using a microscope to analyze vaginal discharge. Metronidazole (Flagyl) is used to treat the infection. Since it is usually acquired through sexual transmission, your partner should be treated to prevent reinfection.

What is PID?

PID, or pelvic inflammatory disease, is a pelvic infection of the uterus, fallopian tubes, and ovaries. It is more serious than the vaginal infec-

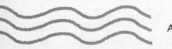

tions described in the previous section. Infection involving the uterus, tubes, and ovaries can create adhesions that produce infertility, tubal pregnancy, or chronic pelvic pain. Severe PID may even develop into a pelvic abscess (collection of pus) that requires drainage or more aggressive surgery. The organisms that cause PID can also produce complications in pregnancy. They can induce miscarriage, preterm labor, or preterm rupture of the membranes. The baby of an infected mother can develop conjunctivitis (an eye infection) or pneumonia.

PID usually begins as an infection of the cervix caused by either gonorrhea or chlamydia (or both), which are sexually transmitted organisms. Cervical infection may produce a discharge from the cervix, but commonly it has no associated symptoms. If untreated, the infection can spread into the uterus and through the fallopian tubes. The most common symptom experienced once the infection has ascended is pelvic pain. If the infection is severe, fever, chills, nausea, and vomiting may accompany it. Other symptoms associated with PID include yellowish vaginal discharge, painful urination, and abnormal vaginal bleeding. These other symptoms, without accompanying pelvic pain, however, are more likely related to other gynecologic disorders. Other possible sites of infection include the rectum (through anal intercourse), the urethra (because of its proximity to the vagina), and the mouth (through oral sex).

When your doctor suspects the presence of PID, he or she will perform a pelvic examination. If you have PID, your pelvic examination will be painful. However, your gynecologist cannot make an accurate assessment without performing this examination. A pelvic ultrasound may also be ordered to detect other possible causes for pelvic pain (such as ovarian cysts and tumors) or the presence of a pelvic abscess. Other laboratory evaluation includes bloodwork and a urinalysis or urine culture to rule out a bladder infection as the source of your pain.

PID is treated with antibiotics that will eliminate both gonorrhea and chlamydia, which frequently coexist. The duration of treatment will vary depending on the severity of the infection. If the infection is mild, you will be treated as an outpatient. It is critical that you complete your entire course of antibiotics. It is tempting to stop treatment once you feel better. However, incomplete treatment can result in persistent infection. You may be admitted to the hospital if you have one of the following conditions:

- Severe infection (as evidenced by the amount of tenderness present, the level of your fever, and your white blood cell count — the cells that fight infections)
- Nausea and vomiting
- A pelvic abscess

When admitted, you will receive intravenous antibiotics. Once it is apparent that the infection is responding to the antibiotics, you will be discharged and can complete the antibiotics at home. If there is an abscess, it may have to be drained by insertion of a catheter or by surgery.

If your partner has signs of infection, such as penile discharge or burning, avoid sex until his problem is evaluated. If it is determined that he has either gonorrhea or chlamydia, you must also be evaluated and treated. Similarly, if you are diagnosed with either infection, he also needs to be treated. Abstain from sexual contact until both of you have completed the entire course of antibiotics and your doctor has determined that your infection has disappeared. If it is possible that you contracted the infection from someone other than your current partner, that person must also be notified and sent for evaluation. If you are treated for either gonorrhea or chlamydia, your doctor may suggest undergoing tests for other sexually transmitted diseases.

Is there any good news about this disease? Yes — it's preventable. Until you have a mutually monogamous relationship — lasting for years, not months — condoms should be used every time you have intercourse, even if you are using other contraceptives. (See page 36 for an in-depth look at condoms). If your partner won't use a condom, use the female condom (Reality). If he still refuses, ditch him. That may seem drastic, but your health is more important than his ego.

How can I tell the difference between a bladder infection and other pelvic infections?

Since the bladder is located next to your reproductive organs, it can be difficult to distinguish bladder problems from vaginal or uterine infections. Bladder infections, also called cystitis, are fairly common in women. The urethral opening is located immediately above the vaginal opening, making it easy for vaginal bacteria to enter the bladder.

You may have pelvic pain right above your pubic bone associated with a bladder infection. More typical symptoms include the following:

- *Urinary urgency:* It seems that you have to race to the bathroom.
- *Frequency:* You experience a marked increase in frequency of urination.
- *Dysuria:* You feel pain or burning with urination.

You may have only one of the symptoms or all three. If you see blood in the urine, don't panic. Bloody urine is common with bladder infections. The diagnosis of cystitis is obtained by urinalysis or urine culture. Treatment consists of antibiotics. Whenever possible, a urine culture should be obtained before starting antibiotics to confirm the diagnosis and to show which bacterium is causing the infection.

Occasional bladder infections should not be alarming. However, if they don't seem to respond to the antibiotics or occur more than three times per year, you should consider seeing a urologist for further evaluation.

Do people still get syphilis?

At one time in history, syphilis was extremely prevalent. With the arrival of penicillin, the number of cases decreased dramatically. However, it remains a dangerous sexually transmitted infection.

Syphilis starts as a single, painless sore (in contrast to the herpes sore, which is painful), called a chancre. Common sites of infection include the genitalia, anus, and mouth. The chancre exists for one to five weeks and then disappears without a trace. If the mucous membranes (which line the mouth, the vagina, and the anus) or broken skin of a sexual partner contacts the chancre, the infection will be transmitted. In women, the chancre is often hidden in the vagina, preventing early detection of the disease. If it goes undetected in this early stage, the disease will reappear as a rash, often accompanied by a flulike illness. The disease then undergoes a period of latency with no symptoms. It can remain latent or reappear years later, causing serious problems with the heart, blood vessels, and nervous system.

The diagnosis of syphilis is usually made through a blood test. If a chancre is present, the organism can be detected by microscopic analysis of fluid from the chancre. Treatment with antibiotics will cure the disease in its early stages. More advanced disease may be difficult to eradicate.

Syphilis can be transmitted during pregnancy from the mother to her fetus. The infection can cause miscarriage, stillbirth, and developmental problems for the baby. Because of this, all pregnant women should have a blood test for syphilis early in pregnancy. If syphilis is detected early, treatment can be instituted, thereby protecting the baby.

When an individual is diagnosed with syphilis, all current and past sexual partners must be examined and tested. Testing for other sexually transmitted diseases should also be performed.

Your best protection against syphilis is to avoid sexual contact with multiple partners. Condoms afford some protection, but only if the chancre is covered by the condom. Examination of a potential sex partner will also reveal a chancre or, for that matter, herpetic blisters, ulcerations, or genital warts. If you see any skin lesions, abstain from sexual contact until the potential partner has been evaluated by a physician.

I have bumps that feel like warts. What are they?

You may be feeling genital warts, but other structures are often confused with warts. It is common to find pimples or cysts on the external genitalia. Sweat glands and sebaceous glands (glands that secrete an oily substance) are located just under the skin. When the ducts of these glands become obstructed, as they often do in the genital region, small pimples or cysts form, which may feel like bumps. You may also feel extra folds of labial skin or remnants of the hymenal ring.

The most common warty lesions of the genitalia are genital warts, also called venereal warts and condylomas. Their formation is induced by a virus called HPV, or human papillomavirus. This sexually transmitted virus infects the vulva, vagina, and cervix. The transmission of this virus has become epidemic, with over 100,000 new cases every year. Infection with HPV (not to be confused with HIV, the virus associated with AIDS) is often asymptomatic and transmitted without the awareness of an infected individual. The warts may be seen within weeks of the infection or even years later. It is difficult to pinpoint the actual date of the initial infection for that reason. You may be the first person to detect the warts, or they may be discovered during a routine gynecologic examination.

Once discovered, warts are treated in a variety of ways. Doctors commonly use one of two chemicals, podophyllin or trichloroacetic acid (TCA), to destroy the warts. If podophyllin is applied, it should be washed off after a period of time (usually within four to six hours) to avoid excess burning. Podophyllin is applied to external warts but not to vaginal or cervical warts. It is not used during pregnancy because of concern that it might cause harm to the fetus. Repeated applications may be required. A podophyllin preparation (Condylox) is also available by prescription for self-application. The solution is applied to the warts with a cotton-tipped applicator for three days, followed by four days without the medication. This one-week cycle may be repeated up to four times. A new topical cream, called Aldara, has received approval for treatment of external and perianal warts. Aldara has no direct antiviral effects but appears to increase the body's local immune response. Patients apply Aldara cream to warts once every other day, three days a week, until the warts are gone or for up to 16 weeks. Use these regimens only with the supervision of your doctor to ensure proper application.

Efudex (fluorouracil) cream is sometimes used to treat vaginal warts. The cream is inserted with an applicator. Great care must be taken to keep Efudex from touching the external skin of the labia and vulva. It can produce severe inflammation and ulceration. Some physicians recommend covering the labia and vulva with petroleum jelly to protect them against cream that may leak from the vagina.

Interferon is another drug used in the treatment of genital warts. Interferons are naturally occurring proteins that the body produces to fight viruses. In this regimen, extra interferon is administered to help the body fight the HPV virus. Interferon can be given intramuscularly or injected directly into the warts by your physician.

Other treatments for genital warts include these:

- *Cryotherapy:* freezing the warts
- *Cautery:* burning the warts
- *Laser:* vaporizing the warts with a high-energy beam
- *Excision:* surgically removing the warts

The best type of treatment is determined by the number, size, and location of the warts. If there are just a few, chemical treatment is usually chosen. If the warts are numerous, large, or resistant to medical treatment, a more aggressive approach is undertaken. Sometimes these procedures can be performed in the doctor's office under local anesthesia. Others may require general anesthesia in an operating room as outpatient surgery.

The most significant feature of HPV virus is its linkage to the development of cervical, vaginal, and vulvar cancer. The virus can cause changes in these genital areas that are potentially precancerous. If you have a history of genital warts or are at increased risk for acquiring HPV virus, regular Pap smears are essential. Your doctor may also want to examine your vagina, vulva, and cervix under magnification, using an instrument called a colposcope. With regular Pap smears, precancerous changes can be detected and treated before they progress. This topic is discussed further in chapters 9 and 11.

Genital warts tend to increase in size during pregnancy. Sometimes they can be treated during pregnancy. If they are extensive, though, the doctor may wait until after delivery to treat them, since the HPV virus does not adversely effect the progress and development of the pregnancy.

The frustrating aspect of genital warts is that recurrence is common. Although the warts have been treated, the HPV virus remains in the surrounding "normal" tissue and can induce the formation of new warts. In contrast to bacteria, viruses cannot be eliminated by antibiotics. With repeated treatment, however, you should eventually be able to eradicate recurrent warts.

If you have genital warts, your partner should also be evaluated. Usually this is done by a urologist, a doctor that treats problems involv-

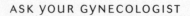

ing the male genitalia. Previous partners should also be notified, if possible. If you suspect that you or your partner may have genital warts, avoid sexual contact until the warts have been treated and completely removed. Although using condoms during sex decreases the risk of transmitting the warts, it doesn't eliminate it.

Receiving the diagnosis of genital warts can be quite disconcerting. Try to remember that this is an extremely common infection. Although HPV virus can induce abnormalities of the cervix, vagina, and vulva, it is almost always detectable with regular exams and is treated easily. The virus and warts do not infect the uterine cavity, fallopian tubes, or ovaries. There is no adverse effect on fertility. The virus resides locally and creates no problems elsewhere in the body.

What is that painful sore down there?

Painful blisters and ulcerations involving the external genitalia may represent a herpes infection. These may occur in conjunction with other infections, so examination and laboratory tests are necessary to obtain an accurate diagnosis. Herpes is a virus that produces blisters and open sores. It commonly infects the genital area, usually through direct sexual contact with an infected partner. Other areas that may be infected include the buttocks, fingers, mouth, and eyes. Two types of herpes commonly cause these infections. Herpes simplex type 1 usually causes oral herpetic lesions, more commonly referred to as fever blisters or cold sores. Herpes simplex type 2 more commonly causes genital herpes. Either type of virus can infect the genitalia. Infection is acquired from active virus found in the blisters or ulcerations. Transmission is usually through one of the following mechanisms:

- Direct contact of your genitalia with the active lesions of a partner
- Autoinoculation — spread of the virus by your touching an active lesion (such as a fever blister) and transferring it to the genitalia
- Oral sex with a partner with oral herpes

No evidence suggests that the virus is acquired from toilet seats, hot tubs, or swimming pools.

The initial infection, also called the primary infection, is likely to be the most severe. Blisters appear, often in groups, at the infected site. The blisters open, forming painful ulcerations. A primary infection may also cause flulike symptoms including fever, fatigue, and muscular aches. Swollen structures in the groin areas represent enlarged lymph nodes. Urination can be painful as urine touches the open sores. The doctor diagnoses herpes by culturing the fluid in the blisters or ulcerations.

Even without treatment, the open lesions dry up and gradually disappear over several weeks. However, most doctors will prescribe an antiviral medication. The most commonly used medication is acyclovir (Zovirax). Recently, two additional medications, famciclovir (Famvir) and valacyclovir (Valtrex), have received approval for the treatment of genital herpes. All of these medications shorten the amount of time required for the lesions to disappear. They are administered orally or as an ointment applied directly to the lesions. Using a blow dryer several times daily keeps the lesions dry and helps them disappear more quickly.

If your lesions cause painful urination, consider voiding in a sitz bath. If the pain associated with the infection is not controlled with over-the-counter analgesics, ask your doctor to prescribe a stronger pain reliever. If you must touch the lesions, use a glove or finger cot (a latex sleeve that slides over a finger to protect it). Also wash your hands thoroughly whenever you may have come in contact with a lesion. Use separate washcloths and towels for bathing while the lesions are present. If you share a bed, wear pajamas while the infection is active. There is no need to wash your clothes or bed linens separately.

Antiviral medications can't clear up the virus completely. After the initial infection, the virus recedes into the nerve cells that supply sensation to the affected area. If the virus becomes reactivated, a recurrence, or secondary infection, will occur. Recurrences appear in the location of the primary infection. However, the lesions are fewer and less severe. Secondary infections usually disappear within a week, often lasting only three to five days. Antiviral medications are of limited benefit in secondary infections because of their short duration. Most recurrences follow the primary infection by 3 to 12 months. Many women never have a recurrence. Others get an outbreak many years after the initial infection. Recurrences are more common during times of stress or fatigue and when the body is fighting another infection, such as a cold or flu. Sometimes there is forewarning in the form of tingling or itching at the site of the recurrence before the lesions appear.

If you get frequent or severe outbreaks, you may be a candidate for taking antiviral medication as a preventive measure. Daily administration of an antiviral medication can significantly decrease the frequency and severity of recurrent outbreaks. The medications are usually tolerated well, and serious adverse reactions are uncommon.

Recurrences during pregnancy are fairly common. They do not pose any harm to the developing baby or interfere with the pregnancy. However, active lesions at the time of birth are a cause for concern. Contact with lesions during delivery can produce serious problems for the baby, including skin infection, blindness, damage to the nervous system, and even death. If signs of a herpetic infection appear near the end of your pregnancy, contact your obstetrician immediately. If an active infection exists when you go into labor or when your membranes rupture (signaled by a gush of fluid), the doctor will deliver the baby by cesarean section to avoid exposing the baby to the herpes virus. Most women with a history of herpes will not have active lesions at the time of delivery and can undergo normal vaginal delivery without concern.

Some studies indicate that herpes increases the risk of getting cervical cancer. Recently this conclusion has been questioned, but you should still get Pap smears once or twice yearly if you have herpes.

The best way to reduce the chance of getting herpes is to avoid sexual contact with anyone who has active herpetic lesions. Condoms do not reliably prevent transmission of the virus, since they do not provide complete coverage of the external genitalia. You must have open communication with your sexual partner. You have to directly ask him if he has ever noticed blisters or sores on his genitalia. If you or your partner has herpes, avoid sex until any scabs have disappeared. If either of you has a "fever blister," avoid contact with the sore — no kissing, touching the mouth, or oral-genital contact — until the lesion has completely disappeared for several days.

For more information concerning herpes, contact the following:

PELVIC INFECTIONS

Herpes Resource Center
American Social Health Association
P.O. Box 13827
Research Triangle Park, NC 27709
www.herpes.com

National Herpes Hotline
(800) 230-6039 (for information)
(919) 361-8488 (for counseling)

Can women get AIDS?

AIDS, or acquired immunodeficiency syndrome, has been associated with male homosexuality, intravenous drug abuse, and blood transfusions. Many people are unaware (or have not accepted) that HIV (human immunodeficiency virus) is transmitted through heterosexual encounters. Heterosexual women constitute a rapidly growing sector within the AIDS population. Accepting this and understanding how to prevent HIV transmission are critical.

HIV is transmitted through intimate contact with the infected body fluids (usually semen or blood) of another person. It is acquired through any of the following mechanisms:

- Sharing the needle of a drug abuser infected with HIV

- Having sex with a person who is infected

- Receiving a blood product contaminated with HIV

Blood transfusions received before 1985 carried a greater risk of HIV contamination. Since then, blood banks have routinely screened their supplies for HIV, and the risk is relatively low. However, if you plan to undergo surgery, ask your doctor if you can give your own blood or designate a blood donor prior to the surgery.

You cannot contract the HIV virus through casual contact with an infected individual. It is not transmitted from sharing items with an infected person (including food, drinks, bathing facilities, pools, and hot tubs). It is not contracted through kissing an infected individual or contacting his or her sweat or tears.

AIDS does not develop immediately after HIV infection. The HIV virus attacks the immune system, and it may be months or years before symptoms develop from the virus. Eventually, though, the infected person becomes weaker and develops infections and unusual types of cancer. When these occur, the diagnosis of AIDS is made. Many people die from AIDS within a few years. Currently there is no cure for HIV infection, although some drugs can decrease the effects of the virus. There is also no vaccine in current use to prevent the transmission of HIV.

Prevention of HIV infection is accomplished by avoiding activities that are associated with high transmission (intravenous drug abuse, anal intercourse) and refraining from sexual contact with men who are at high risk of being infected (intravenous drug users, bisexual men, men with a history of multiple sexual partners). Latex condoms, used appropriately, prevent the transmission of AIDS during sex.

If you contract a different sexually transmitted disease, it is prudent to undergo testing for HIV. If you are in a high-risk group, you should also be tested, particularly if you anticipate becoming pregnant. As many as one third of all infected women will transmit the infection to their babies, either during pregnancy or delivery. Women with HIV who breast-feed their infants can also transmit the virus to them. Testing is performed on a blood sample. Most health care centers will provide HIV testing confidentially. Either your doctor or a health care provider at the testing site should counsel patients before and after the test. The blood test for HIV does not register as positive immediately after infection with the virus. Therefore, it is advisable to take a second test approximately six months after the initial screening.

If you test positive, all current and past sexual partners must be notified and tested. Further sexual activity must be undertaken only with the use of latex condoms and with the informed consent of your partner. Other contraceptives should be used with the condoms to prevent pregnancy. HIV-positive individuals should never donate blood or plasma or register as an organ donor. All health care providers must be informed of your HIV-positive status, including your dentist. Objects that may be contaminated with blood, such as toothbrushes and razors, should not be shared with others. If you acquire HIV, it is important for you to seek a physician with experience in caring for AIDS patients.

PELVIC INFECTIONS

You should also consult with a therapist or join a support group to help you cope.

Can you get hepatitis through sex?

You bet! Most people think of hepatitis as a disease acquired through food. Indeed, some types of hepatitis are contracted in this manner. Hepatitis type B, however, can be transmitted through body fluids such as blood, semen, vaginal secretions, and saliva. It can therefore be transmitted through sexual intercourse. It can also be transmitted through contact with the blood of an infected individual or by sharing needles with drug abusers.

Hepatitis B is a virus that infects the liver, causing fatigue, nausea, abdominal pain, and jaundice (yellowish pigmentation of the skin). In most cases, the body forms antibodies that attack the virus, and the infection is resolved. However, some individuals develop a chronic form of the disease (chronic hepatitis) and are contagious to those who contact their body fluids. Some people infected with the virus never get sick but remain contagious "carriers" of the virus. Pregnant women can transmit the virus to the unborn child, who may develop hepatitis or become a carrier. People who have chronic hepatitis or are carriers have an increased risk of dying from liver failure or liver cancer.

Diagnosis of hepatitis is made through a blood test. Testing can detect whether you have ever had hepatitis and if you can transmit the virus to others. No treatment can eradicate the virus, but a vaccine can prevent you from getting it. Vaccination is essential if you

- are single and sexually active
- have multiple sex partners
- live with someone who has hepatitis or is a carrier
- have contracted another sexually transmitted disease
- inject illegal drugs
- work in the health care field
- work in any field that increases your risk of contact with body fluids
- have a disease that requires you to receive blood products

A woman who is pregnant should be tested. If she tests positive, other tests can be performed to ensure that liver function is normal. At birth her baby can be given hepatitis B immune globulin (antibodies) to fight the virus. The baby will also be vaccinated. This regimen is 95 percent effective at preventing infection of the newborn.

The risk of contracting hepatitis through sex is decreased with the use of latex condoms. The best preventive measure, though, is vaccination. Vaccination of all teenagers is recommended by many health care providers.

If I get a sexually transmitted disease, should I be tested for others?

Sexually transmitted diseases (STDs) often coexist. If you have one infection, there is a possibility that other STDs have been transmitted to you, even if they show no signs or symptoms. If your doctor diagnoses a STD, he or she will often collect cultures and order bloodwork to screen you for other diseases. You should also consider screening for STDs if you have been involved in one or more of these high-risk behaviors:

- Sexual activity with more than one partner
- Sexual activity without using condoms
- Sexual contact with a person who has developed an STD

Why can't the gynecologist cure my infection?

Some sexually transmitted diseases, such as chlamydia and gonorrhea, are curable with antibiotics because they are caused by bacteria that the medication kills. There is no cure, however, for sexually transmitted viruses: herpes, HPV, HIV, hepatitis. The immune system mounts a defense against the virus that may contain it or reduce its activity, but often the virus remains and springs up later. Medications can help reduce the activity of the virus, but none can rid the body of the virus.

Dealing with a chronic infection is frustrating and depressing. Advances in genetic technology and pharmacology should eventually provide us with the cure for these infections. Work is also under way to develop vaccines to prevent transmission of these viruses. Try to maintain a positive outlook. Help is on the way!

What can I do to avoid getting a sexually transmitted disease?

After reading this chapter, you're probably considering a major change in lifestyle, perhaps enlisting as a novice at the nearest convent. That may be a little too drastic a solution, although abstinence has merit. The only sure way to avoid STDs is to avoid sex. Ideally, you should proceed with sexual intimacy only when you have a long-standing mutually monogamous relationship. At least you should try to limit the number of your sexual partners. Ask a potential sexual partner about his past and any signs of possible infection (sores, warts, discharge). If there is any question of a current or prior STD, he should be examined. Abstain from sex until he has been evaluated, and be adamant about this. If his history includes prior sex partners, strongly consider HIV testing. Consider examining a potential sex partner before intercourse (you can combine this with placing a condom on the penis). Look for warts, blisters, and ulcerations. Always use condoms! When using a male condom, use the latex type. Natural "skin" condoms do not offer adequate protection against STDs. An alternative is the female condom, but it is not as well tested for STD prevention. (Refer to chapter 3 for further information on condoms.)

How do I cope emotionally when I discover that I have a sexually transmitted disease?

Society has promoted the concept that sexually transmitted diseases should be worn like a "scarlet letter." This attitude implies that one must be flagrantly promiscuous and devoid of morality to contract such a disease. This certainly is not true. Because viruses such as herpes and HPV (human papillomavirus, which causes genital warts) are not yet curable, their prevalence in the general population is tremendous. You can contract these even with limited sexual encounters. Unfortunately, the prevailing attitude may make you feel embarrassed and ashamed when diagnosed with a sexually transmitted disease. You may feel angry at yourself or the partner who gave you the infection — or even at the

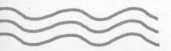

entire male population. While working through these issues, keep in mind the following points:

- Blaming yourself is not constructive. In many cases, there is nothing you could have done to prevent catching the virus. Obsessing about the past won't help you develop a positive approach to dealing with your infection.

- Openly discuss your situation with your partner. If he was not honest with you regarding a history of herpes or HPV, you have every right to feel angry and betrayed. You should question whether it is wise to continue a relationship with a man who cannot be honest even when your health is at stake. However, keep in mind that sexually transmitted diseases can be asymptomatic, and your partner may have been unaware that he was infected. He may have acquired the infection months, or even years, prior to transmitting it to you. Likewise, you may have acquired the infection before your relationship with him. If both of you are honest and unaware of the origin of the infection, assigning blame only serves to destroy your relationship.

- If a marriage (or other mutually monogamous relationship) has existed for many years and a sexually transmitted infection appears, you should suspect that extramarital sex has occurred. If this is a possibility, confront your husband. Extramarital affairs often reflect serious problems within a relationship. You should definitely consider couples counseling.

- If you are in a new relationship and have a history of herpes or HPV, you must discuss this with your partner prior to sexual intimacy. You need to communicate openly with him. If he loves you, this should not be an insurmountable obstacle to deepening your relationship. Make sure he understands the facts about your condition, and help clear up any misconceptions he may harbor about it. A joint visit to your gynecologist may help.

- If you are having trouble coping, consider enrolling in a support group. Ask your doctor and call surrounding hospitals to see if there is a support group in your area. There may also be a listing in the phone directory in the "guide to human services" section. Your county medical society may also be able to direct you to a group. At support groups, you will find other women who share your feelings and are struggling with the same issues. Sometimes comfort is gained in discovering that you are not alone. Group members can share approaches that have enabled them to deal with the infection and emotional distress.

- Abstaining from sex during times of active infection doesn't mean you can't share intimate moments with your partner. Spending quiet time talking, kissing, and cuddling can enable you to show affection even during bouts of active infection. There is no risk in being close as long as there is no direct contact with lesions.

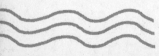

6 Why Can't I Get Pregnant?

I've been trying to get pregnant for six months. Does this mean I have a problem?

Don't jump to conclusions. Women sometimes get so consumed with preventing pregnancy that they assume it will occur the first month they stop using contraception. In reality, you only have a 20 percent chance of conceiving in any single cycle. Most gynecologists do not suspect an infertility problem until a couple has tried to conceive for one year without success. You should wait at least that long before seeking an infertility evaluation. If you want to increase your chances of success, you can time intercourse to happen just before you ovulate.

Of course, everything is relative. One year seems like an eternity as you're approaching age 40 and hearing the tick-tock, tick-tock of that infernal biological clock. In your later reproductive years, after age 35, starting an evaluation after six months of timed intercourse is reasonable.

When is the best time in my cycle for conception?

If your sex life is flourishing, you'll be tempted to answer, "All the time!" However enjoyable that may be, successful conception is limited to a specific point in your cycle. The greatest chances of success occur two to three days before ovulation through 24 hours after ovulation. The section on natural family planning on page 35 shows how to determine your day of ovulation. You can use this information to enhance your chances of conception, as well as to prevent it. Try to have sexual intercourse every other day, beginning two to four days prior to anticipated ovulation. It is best not to have intercourse every day, as this may

FERTILITY PROBLEMS

decrease your partner's sperm count. He should also refrain from masturbation for several days prior to your first scheduled sexual encounter.

Do I need to see an infertility specialist?

You have tried to conceive for a year without success. What do you do now? That depends on the background and philosophy of your gynecologist. Many have the qualifications and interest to start your infertility evaluation. The initial tests are fairly basic and can be performed competently by a general gynecologist. You may feel more comfortable remaining with a doctor you know, rather than starting with a new, unfamiliar one. Also, a gynecologist's fees are generally lower than those of an infertility specialist. However, the evaluation may proceed more expeditiously with a specialist. If the initial tests do not find an obvious source of your problem, you would do best to consult a specialist. Ask your gynecologist if the tests will have to be repeated if you are referred to a specialist. If so, you are better off seeing an infertility specialist from the start.

What is a BBT chart?

The BBT (basal body temperature) chart reflects your ovarian function. Immediately upon awakening each day, record your temperature on a special chart provided by your doctor. To keep a precise record, this must be done before you begin any other activity. (Well, OK, you can breathe — but nothing else!) You can purchase a basal body thermometer, which is easy to read, at your local pharmacy. After ovulation, your ovary produces progesterone that induces a temperature rise of one-half to one degree. By analyzing the chart, your doctor can determine if you have ovulated and the day of ovulation. The doctor also uses your BBT chart when planning the timing of certain tests.

How can the gynecologist tell if I have a problem?

A common misconception is that a routine pelvic examination will provide your doctor with sufficient information to determine if you have an infertility problem. Most infertility problems require specialized testing. The evaluation can be expensive and time consuming. Some procedures may be uncomfortable (that's what doctors say to avoid the

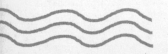

word *painful*). Many tests have to be scheduled at specific times in your cycle. The evaluation often disrupts your daily routines and doesn't exactly enhance the romance of your marriage.

About now you're saying, "Gee, you could be a little more upbeat about this." We apologize. However, it is important to realize that an infertility evaluation is not to be taken lightly. A strong sense of commitment is needed to launch into a potentially long-term, emotionally draining process. With this in mind, let's identify the various sources of infertility. We will describe each problem, the tests required for its detection, and the treatment. (You may want to refer to the illustration of the female reproductive system on page 24.)

Problems with Ovulation If your ovary doesn't release an egg, you won't conceive. In other words, having eggs in your ovaries does not guarantee that you will ovulate. The sperm can fertilize an egg only after it has been released from the ovary. The eggs reside in small fluid-filled structures in the ovaries referred to as follicles. Signals, called gonadotropins, are sent from the pituitary gland (a small gland located at the base of the brain) to stimulate the follicles in the ovary. Normally, each month one of these follicles reaches maturation and ovulates, thereby releasing the egg. The secretion of gonadotropins from the pituitary must be precisely timed, and anything that interferes with it will result in failure to ovulate (called anovulation). Stress or anxiety may temporarily prevent ovulation. Excessive or inadequate weight may also play a role. Numerous medical disorders can have an effect on gonadotropin secretion. The problem may reside within the ovary. The ovary may be congenitally abnormal, may have become resistant to gonadotropins, or may have undergone the effects of early menopause. Many women evidence no apparent reason for failure to ovulate.

Your BBT chart and a progesterone level obtained during the second half of your cycle can determine whether ovulation has occurred. If your BBT chart does not show a rise in temperature and your progesterone level is low, you have not ovulated. A rise in temperature and an elevated progesterone level indicate successful ovulation. Sometimes the progesterone level and BBT chart suggest ovulation, but the ovary still doesn't release an egg, a problem that can be detected by performing ultrasound scans when you are in the middle of your cycle. After the diagnosis of anovulation is established, your doctor will order bloodwork. This helps rule out certain medical disorders, such as thyroid disease, that prevent ovulation.

To stimulate the release of gonadotropins from the pituitary and to induce ovulation, doctors usually first prescribe clomiphene citrate (Clomid or Serophene). Clomiphene causes 80 percent of patients to successfully ovulate, and 40 percent of them conceive. If patients with additional causes of infertility are excluded, the conception rate approaches 80 percent. Clomiphene does not increase the risk of miscarriage and birth defects. The incidence of twins is increased to 5 percent with clomiphene. Multiple births are rare. Potential side effects include hot flushes, abdominal bloating, breast tenderness, mood alteration, nausea, headache, and visual changes. Usually these conditions are transient, and most women tolerate clomiphene well.

Patients who do not respond to clomiphene typically receive a prescription for Pergonal. Pergonal consists of the same gonadotropins normally secreted by the pituitary gland. Injected into the body, they directly stimulate the ovary, inducing follicular maturation. Pergonal is very expensive and has the potential for significant complications. Therefore, it is critical to rule out other causes of infertility prior to its use. Women should be monitored closely while using Pergonal, and it should be administered by an infertility specialist since it can stimulate the formation of cysts in the ovaries, which can rupture.

Multiple pregnancy rates increase by 10 percent or more with use of Pergonal. Most multiple pregnancies — triplets, quadruplets, quintuplets — occur in women who have used Pergonal. Multiple pregnancies may seem exciting, but they are associated with many pregnancy complications, especially premature delivery.

Problems of the Luteal Phase Infertility is not always caused by a failure to ovulate, however. If the second half of the cycle (known as the luteal phase) is either shortened or inadequate, infertility can result. The follicle remaining after ovulation, referred to as the corpus luteum, fails to produce sufficient progesterone. Progesterone prepares the endometrium for implantation of the embryo and supports the early pregnancy. The pregnancy will be unsuccessful if progesterone production is inadequate. The BBT chart suggests a luteal phase disorder if the temperature rise following ovulation is abbreviated. A low progesterone level in the midluteal phase also indicates a luteal deficiency. The doctor may want to perform an endometrial biopsy. After inserting a speculum, he or she introduces a biopsy instrument through the cervix to obtain an endometrial sample. A pathologist interprets the specimen to see if the endometrium has been properly prepared by progesterone.

Luteal phase deficiencies are treated in several ways. The most common approach is to supplement progesterone during the luteal phase. Progesterone is given either orally or via vaginal suppositories. Should conception occur, progesterone is continued during the first trimester to provide support for the early pregnancy. Natural progesterone is not associated with an increased risk of birth defects. A second approach is to stimulate follicular maturation with drugs such as clomiphene, resulting in an improved corpus luteum that produces higher progesterone levels.

Tubal Problems Once the egg is released from the ovary, it must travel down the fallopian tube for fertilization and eventual implantation in the uterus (see the illustration on page 92). If the fallopian tubes are closed or scar tissue (adhesions) is interposed between the ovaries and tubes, this is not possible. Conditions that may contribute to tubal blockage or adhesions include severe pelvic infections, IUD use, endometriosis, prior pelvic surgery, tubal pregnancies, and appendicitis.

The hysterosalpingogram (HSG) is a radiographic test used to see whether the tubes are blocked. It is scheduled in the first half of the cycle, at least several days after menstruation has ceased. After inserting a speculum, the doctor places a small catheter into the cervix and injects a contrast dye into the uterus and tubes. X-rays are taken. If the tubes are patent (open), dye emerges from the tubes. If they are obstructed, the doctor notes the location of the blockage. The HSG also provides information regarding uterine abnormalities, such as polyps, fibroids, or an unusually shaped uterus. Laparoscopy (see page 21) is also employed if the results of the HSG are not clear.

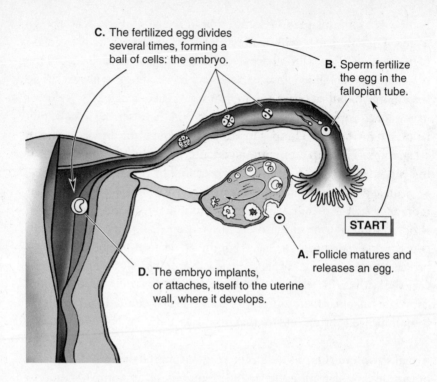

C. The fertilized egg divides several times, forming a ball of cells: the embryo.

B. Sperm fertilize the egg in the fallopian tube.

START

A. Follicle matures and releases an egg.

D. The embryo implants, or attaches, itself to the uterine wall, where it develops.

Intrauterine disorders are evaluated by hysteroscopy. The doctor inserts a telescopic instrument through the cervix, allowing him or her to see inside the uterus. Intrauterine fibroids, polyps, and adhesions can be removed through the hysteroscope. Some uterine malformations can also be corrected. (Refer to chapter 9 for more detailed information on uterine disorders and hysteroscopy.)

There are several methods of correcting tubal blockage. If most of the tube is healthy, your doctor may elect to remove the obstructed portion and reattach the remaining sections of tube. This is a surgical procedure referred to as tubal reanastomosis. If the blockage is located at the cornua (where the tube joins the uterus), the doctor may choose to reimplant the tube through an opening created in the uterus. Blockage at the end of the tube (the fimbria) is repaired by releasing the adhesions that encase the tube or by creating a new opening. In some circumstances a semiflexible wire called a stent can be passed through a tubal obstruction by using the hysteroscope.

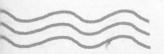

If your tubes are beyond salvage, you still have the option of in vitro fertilization (IVF). In this procedure, your eggs are removed from the ovaries during laparoscopy or with a needle that is directed by ultrasonic guidance. The eggs are fertilized with sperm in a laboratory. The fertilized egg divides several times, forming a ball of cells called the embryo, which is placed directly into the uterus through the vagina. You have a one in five chance of success with each in vitro attempt. GIFT (gamete intrafallopian transfer) and ZIFT (zygote intrafallopian transfer) are variations of IVF that involve transferring eggs directly into a healthy portion of tube. IVF is very expensive, although its cost has been decreasing as more centers develop IVF capabilities. Before choosing a center for IVF, investigate the cost and the success rate of the facility.

Cervical Problems Sperm must pass through the cervix to fertilize the egg. Cervical mucus changes prior to ovulation, becoming abundant, watery, thin, and clear. The quality of the mucus affects the sperm's ability to enter the uterus.

The doctor evaluates mucus by using a postcoital test. Immediately prior to ovulation, the woman is asked to have intercourse and then to undergo an examination. The doctor inserts the speculum and gathers mucus from the cervix. If there are signs of infection, the doctor obtains cultures. The postcoital test also gives the doctor an opportunity to assess the ability of the sperm to survive in the mucus. Sperm are assessed for their number, shape, and ability to move. If the sperm appear normal during a semen analysis (see the next question), but not on the postcoital test, factors hostile to sperm must be present in the mucus. These may include poor mucus, infection, presence of lubricants (K-Y jelly and Surgilube can kill sperm), and antibodies that may be hostile to sperm.

Identifying the culprit is the first step in responding to an abnormal postcoital test. Treatment depends on the cause of the problem. Infections are eliminated with antibiotics. Poor-quality mucus is treated with estrogen prior to ovulation. If sperm appear not to move despite good-quality mucus and a normal semen analysis, additional tests may show presence of antibodies (proteins secreted by the immune system that attack anything foreign that invades the body), which may affect the sperm. When viruses and bacteria that threaten health are present, this immune defense is desirable. It's not so desirable when directed against your husband's sperm, however.

When cervical factors causing infertility cannot be corrected, the cervix is bypassed by using intrauterine insemination. The sperm are introduced directly into the intrauterine cavity, using a small catheter.

What about my husband? Should he be checked?

"It doesn't seem fair that I have to go through all of this."

You're right. However, he doesn't completely escape. Your husband must undergo semen analysis, although a normal postcoital test may make this unnecessary. Now it's his time to endure a little embarrassment. After abstaining from sex for several days, he provides a semen specimen by masturbation. It must be collected in a clean container and brought to the laboratory within one hour. The semen is examined to determine how many sperm it contains, whether they move, and whether their shape is normal. The semen is also checked for signs of infection. Abnormalities can be produced by any of the following conditions:

- Past history of mumps, sexually transmitted diseases, surgery near the reproductive organs, or testicular injury
- Use of certain drugs, including some antibiotics, chemotherapy drugs, marijuana, tobacco, and alcohol
- Exposure to radiation
- Excessive heat caused by tight underwear, hot tubs, baths, and saunas
- Varicose veins in the scrotum
- Genetic abnormalities
- Hormonal disorders such as thyroid disease or decreased testosterone production
- Infection
- Structural malformations of the sex organs

- Retrograde ejaculation, in which semen is released backward into the bladder instead of exiting through the penis

Male infertility is usually evaluated and treated by a urologist. You may also be able to locate a physician in your area that specializes in male infertility.

Why does the doctor want to perform a laparoscopy?

If no source for infertility is found on initial testing, your doctor will want to perform a laparoscopy. Adhesions and endometriosis (refer to chapter 8) are two causes of infertility that cannot be accurately diagnosed by scans but must be examined directly through laparoscopy (see page 21). Endometriosis may be discovered through this procedure, and pelvic adhesions are easily discernible. If an HSG was not previously performed, or the results were not clear, dye is injected to exclude the possibility that the fallopian tubes are blocked. Adhesions and endometriosis are then treated by employing laparoscopic techniques.

What is artificial insemination?

Occasionally, conception is enhanced by artificially placing sperm in direct proximity to the uterus. If your husband's sperm count is poor, specimens can be pooled and then placed in the vagina, cervix, or uterus. This is referred to as AIH (artificial insemination of husband) or artificial insemination of sperm. It is also used when the semen is normal but cannot be properly deposited in the vagina because of retrograde or premature ejaculation. The specimen is placed near the uterus with either a catheter or cervical cap, and the woman must then lie down, with hips elevated, for 20 to 30 minutes.

If your husband's sperm quality is very poor and cannot be improved, artificial insemination of donor sperm (AID) should be considered. As a rule, the identity of the donor should be unknown to the prospective parents. It is critical for donor semen to be screened to exclude sexually transmittable diseases. Donors should be questioned with respect to family history, genetic disorders, and any past exposure to drugs or chemicals that might increase the risk of birth defects. Your doctor can provide you with details regarding the screening process used for AID specimens.

I hear that infertility drugs cause ovarian cancer. Is that true?

One study indicated an increased risk of getting ovarian cancer with previous use of infertility medications, but flaws with the design of this study make these results questionable. Other investigators have not found an association of ovarian cancer with fertility drugs (clomiphene or Pergonal).

Although it seems reasonable that drugs that induce ovulation might increase the risk of developing ovarian cancer, since oral contraceptives, which inhibit ovulation, decrease the risk, you must remember that these drugs are used for a relatively short period of time. If there is a small risk, it may be offset if you successfully achieve pregnancy, which confers a degree of protection against ovarian cancer.

At this point, clomiphene and Pergonal can be used when necessary to induce ovulation. They should not be taken casually, and the duration of use should be limited.

Why do I feel as if I'm riding an emotional roller coaster?

Infertility can play havoc with your emotions. Discovering that you have an infertility problem can elicit feelings of anger, denial, guilt, grief, and isolation. You assume that pregnancy will occur naturally. When it doesn't, your self-esteem can be shattered. Additional pressure may come from friends and family: "Your sister Judy just had her third baby. When are you going to start?" Avoiding contact with siblings and friends who have already conceived may lead to social isolation.

The infertility evaluation itself is laden with emotional upheaval. Many tests and procedures require scheduled intercourse, which zaps the romance out of marriage. Hopeful anticipation accompanies each attempt at conception. This is soon replaced with frustration and despair if the attempt is not successful. Counseling or therapy with a psychologist may help if you are having trouble coping. You can ask if there is a support group available in your area. If you have trouble finding a support group in your area, contact the national office of RESOLVE

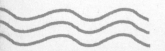

(see page 102). Taking periodic breaks from all the testing for one to three months may also help you cope with the stress.

Throughout the evaluation, your doctor must give you clear appraisals concerning your chances of success. As long as there is a reasonable chance of becoming pregnant, you should persist. Most women who persevere through the infertility evaluation will achieve a successful pregnancy. However, there may come a time when it becomes clear that success is unlikely. At that point, you must try to accept that you may never become pregnant. You can then start investigating alternatives such as adoption.

7 When Something Goes Wrong: Complications of Early Pregnancy

I missed my period and had a positive pregnancy test. Now I'm bleeding. Am I having a miscarriage?

This seems to be a good time to panic, right? Not necessarily. It is common to have light bleeding early in a normal pregnancy. If the bleeding is light, your odds of maintaining the pregnancy are good. If the bleeding is heavy, your chances of success are diminished. When you pass tissue other than blood or clots from the vagina, miscarriage is inevitable.

You should schedule an appointment with your gynecologist at the first sign of bleeding. The doctor will determine your B-HCG (beta-human chorionic gonadotropin) level. B-HCG is a hormone produced by the placenta. The amount of this hormone rises steadily through the first ten weeks of a pregnancy. The value doubles approximately every two days. By comparing sequential values of B-HCG, the doctor can assess the health of the early pregnancy. If the B-HCG level fails to rise appropriately, the pregnancy will not be successful. As long as it rises properly, there is hope of keeping the pregnancy. The doctor may also want to measure a progesterone level, and if it is low, prescribe supplemental progesterone to support the pregnancy. A very low progesterone level suggests that the pregnancy will not survive.

Once the B-HCG reaches a certain level, a pelvic ultrasound scan is done, revealing a pregnancy sac containing an embryo. At this point, or shortly thereafter, a heartbeat should be detectable. If these life signs cannot be discerned, there is no living embryo. As the embryo grows, consecutive studies are done. If growth ceases or the heartbeat stops, the pregnancy is over.

What needs to be done if I'm having a miscarriage?

Once it is determined that pregnancy loss is inevitable, the doctor often recommends a D&E (dilation and evacuation). If the pregnancy was very early, this may not be necessary. The uterus spontaneously expels the nonviable pregnancy completely. After the first few weeks, this is less likely. Your chances of sustaining prolonged, heavy bleeding are substantial, and it's better to evacuate the failed pregnancy by D&E, which is performed as outpatient surgery. After sedation or anesthesia, instruments are placed through the vagina and into the uterus. Nonviable tissue is evacuated from the uterus, thereby allowing it to return to normal. Miscarriage beyond 14 weeks may necessitate an extended D&E or labor-inducing procedure (refer to chapter 3).

Why did I have a miscarriage?

This is one of life's mysterious questions. Unfortunately, most of the time your doctor will not be able to identify the cause of your loss. The mechanisms involved in a developing pregnancy are intricate. Following fertilization, the egg must divide repeatedly and produce perfect duplication of chromosomes (the structures containing your genetic blueprints). A ball of cells forms and implants itself on the inside wall of the uterus and then develops into the placenta and embryo. The placenta must evolve successfully to provide nutrients to the embryo. The cells of the embryo must develop into tissues, and tissues into organs. The complexity of this series of events is almost incomprehensible. If any processes fail, the pregnancy will end. Miscarriage is nature's way of eliminating abnormal pregnancies.

Miscarriages are very common. Twenty percent of all conceptions result in miscarriage. This is important to understand. The tendency is to feel guilty about having one. "Is it something I took (a drink or a medication)? Is it something I did?" Such possible causes are unlikely. Women often feel they are at fault for losing the pregnancy or defective in some way. But in general, the woman is not responsible for the miscarriage.

How long should I wait after a miscarriage before trying again?

This should depend on your emotional state. Some women will want to try again as soon as possible, whereas others need more time for grieving. You should wait at least two menstrual cycles before attempting to conceive again. This permits ample time for your reproductive organs to recover and reestablish a normal ovulatory cycle. You may increase your risk of subsequent miscarriage if you attempt to conceive sooner. Waiting also allows for a period of observation in case you develop a complication from the miscarriage, such as erratic bleeding or infection. Finally, it provides your doctor a better opportunity for dating the pregnancy. If you conceive prior to regaining regular periods, it is harder to establish your estimated "date of confinement," or due date.

I had two miscarriages. Is there something wrong with me?

It is not uncommon to have two successive miscarriages. The odds of that happening are 1 in 25. Three successive miscarriages are considered uncommon and warrant further investigation. Even then, the source of the recurrent pregnancy loss may not be evident. However, it is reasonable to search for one.

Chromosomal aberrations commonly cause miscarriage. Chromosomes are the structures that contain genes, the material encoded with the information that determines a person's constitution. Every cell in the body has an identical set of chromosomes. If there is a failure in the duplication or distribution of the chromosomes during the development of the baby, miscarriage will occur.

Most chromosomal problems are isolated to a specific pregnancy and do not result in repeated pregnancy loss. However, if you or your husband carries a chromosomal irregularity, it may cause recurrent pregnancy loss. This condition can be detected through genetic analysis of chromosomes obtained from cells in the bloodstream (both of you provide a blood specimen). Sometimes genetic analysis can be performed on tissue obtained at the time of the miscarriage. If a chromosomal disturbance is the cause, a genetic counselor can aid you in

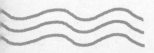

determining your future chances of success and also advise you about genetic studies that might be required during pregnancy.

A fairly common cause for pregnancy loss is progesterone deficiency caused by a luteal phase disorder (see page 90). Progesterone prepares the endometrium (the inside lining of the uterus) for implantation of the embryo and subsequently is required for sustaining the pregnancy.

Uterine infection can be associated with repeated miscarriages. To determine whether such a problem exists, cultures of the cervix are collected in the office. Appropriate antibiotics are prescribed if infection is found.

Abnormalities in the contour or shape of the uterine cavity can produce recurrent pregnancy loss. Some of these may be congenital, meaning that the woman was born with the abnormality. Fibroids — benign, smooth muscle tumors that develop in the wall of the uterus and project into the uterine cavity — can interfere with pregnancy, resulting in miscarriage (see page 114). Scar tissue from prior surgery or infections may also cause pregnancy loss. Uterine abnormalities are diagnosed through a hysterosalpingogram (see page 91) or hysteroscopy and are corrected through surgery. Often the surgery can be performed through the hysteroscope, a telescopic instrument introduced through the vagina into the uterus.

Certain medical disorders may increase the risk of miscarriage. These include systemic lupus erythematosus (an autoimmune disorder), thyroid disease, chronic kidney disease, congenital heart disease, and diabetes. A thorough medical history and physical exam, in conjunction with screening bloodwork, will detect these problems. Often conception can be attempted once these conditions are treated or stabilized.

Disorders of the immune system may result in recurrent pregnancy loss. It is natural for the body to treat the baby as something foreign. Normally, the immune system has a mechanism that prevents the body from rejecting the baby, but this may malfunction. In another immune disorder, the body makes antibodies that cause clotting in placental blood vessels. This disorder is treated with low doses of blood thinners (aspirin or heparin) or with potent anti-inflammatory drugs called corticosteroids.

Also, factors under a woman's control may be responsible for recurrent miscarriages. Smoking, heavy alcohol consumption, and illicit drug use all increase the risk of pregnancy loss. Eliminating these habits is critical to sustaining a healthy pregnancy. Exposure to high doses of radiation or toxic chemicals has also been implicated in causing miscarriage.

Recurrent pregnancy loss can be psychologically devastating. From the moment of conception, you begin to prepare yourself mentally and emotionally for pregnancy and childbirth. Failure of the pregnancy can bring grief, guilt, and anger. Feelings of hopelessness and loss may persist long after a miscarriage, only to be compounded when another miscarriage occurs. Only 60 percent of affected couples ever discover the cause for such recurrent loss. Anger at the medical community for not solving this problem is an understandable reaction. If you are having difficulty coping, contact a support group or psychologist. You may also find the book *A Silent Sorrow: Recurrent Pregnancy Loss* by Ingrid Kohn, M.S.W., Perry-Lynn Moffit, and Isabel A. Wilkins (Dell Publishing, 1992) valuable in dealing with these difficult emotions. Finally, take heart in the fact that 60 to 70 percent of women with recurrent loss that has no identifiable cause will ultimately have a successful pregnancy.

National support groups for couples with recurrent pregnancy loss are listed here.

Diane D. Aronson
RESOLVE
1310 Broadway
Somerville, MA 02144-1731
(617) 623-0744
www.resolve.org

Catherine A. Lammert, R.N.
National SHARE Office
St. Joseph Health Center
300 First Capital Drive
St. Charles, MO 63301
(314) 947-6164
www.nationalshareoffice.com

Gail E. Staples, M.P.H.
Pregnancy and Infant Loss Center
1421 E. Wayzata Boulevard
Wayzata, MN 55391
(612) 473-9372

Maureen Connelly
A.M.E.N.D.
4324 Berrywick Terrace
St. Louis, MO 63128
(314) 487-7582

What is a tubal pregnancy?

Fertilization of the egg occurs in the fallopian tube. The fertilized egg divides several times, forming a ball of cells called the embryo. Usually the embryo becomes implanted in the uterus. However, if the fertilized egg cannot reach the uterus, it implants itself in the wall of the tube and begins to grow. (See the illustration on page 104.) This is referred to as a tubal pregnancy. It is the most common form of ectopic pregnancy, meaning one that is not located in the uterus. Other rare forms of ectopic pregnancy include ovarian pregnancy (implanted on the surface of the ovary) and abdominal pregnancy (implanted elsewhere in the abdomen). Tubal pregnancies occur in approximately 1 out of every 50 pregnancies.

Conditions that may obstruct the fallopian tube increase the risk of developing a tubal pregnancy. Pelvic inflammatory disease, endometriosis, and pelvic surgery may produce scar tissue that may interfere with the passage of the fertilized egg to the uterus. A history of infertility or prior tubal pregnancies heightens the risk of this as well. In many cases, the cause of the tubal pregnancy cannot be identified. Sometimes this indicates a congenital defect in the structure or function of the tube.

Tubal pregnancies are very dangerous. Because the fallopian tube is narrow and cannot expand, the pregnancy eventually bursts through the tube, resulting in heavy internal bleeding. If left untreated, this

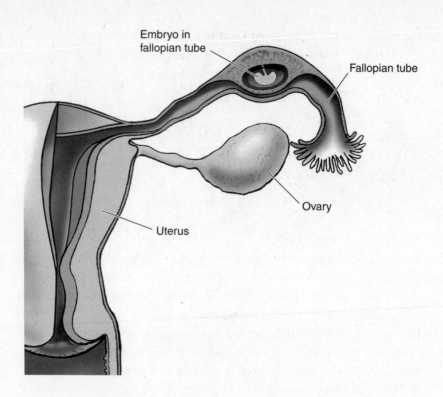

Embryo in
fallopian tube

Fallopian tube

Ovary

Uterus

condition ultimately results in shock, followed by death. Fortunately, symptoms such as pain or abnormal vaginal bleeding raise suspicion and allow the doctor to intervene. Other symptoms include shoulder pain (caused by blood gathering under the diaphragm) and dizziness or faintness caused by blood loss. Tubal pregnancies are never successful. Once this problem is diagnosed, treatment to minimize complications should begin.

I am pregnant and have pain. Do I have a tubal pregnancy?

Have we scared you out of your wits? Thanks to us, every time you get a pain early in pregnancy, you'll be convinced that you have a tubal pregnancy. Actually, many common sources of pain characterize early pregnancy, and most of them are not serious. As the uterus begins to grow, it may cause crampy pain or discomfort. The stretching of the ligaments, the structures that attach the uterus to the pelvic walls, also

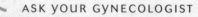

ASK YOUR GYNECOLOGIST

causes discomfort. Usually these types of pain are transient. Cramping and bleeding that occur together are far more likely to represent the threat of a miscarriage than a tubal pregnancy. Pain confined to one side raises more concern. Even then, it may not signify a tubal pregnancy. It is fairly common to develop an ovarian cyst early in pregnancy, and it can cause pain. This cyst derives from the corpus luteum, a normal follicular structure in the ovary. It will resolve spontaneously and requires no treatment.

If you have pelvic pain or bleeding early in pregnancy, don't panic. Call your doctor and ask to be evaluated. If the doctor is concerned after reviewing your history and performing an exam, he or she will obtain an ultrasound scan and check the level of serum B-HCG, the hormone produced by the placenta (see page 98). If the pregnancy is located inside the uterus and no tubal abnormalities are found, no further evaluation is necessary. If the pregnancy cannot be seen in the uterus and the B-HCG level indicates that it should be visible, an ectopic pregnancy must be suspected. If your history includes heavy bleeding or passage of tissue, miscarriage is more likely than an ectopic pregnancy. Sometimes an ultrasound scan clearly shows that the pregnancy is located in the tube. If the doctor is uncertain about the status of your pregnancy, you will be scheduled for laparoscopy. By inserting this telescopic instrument through an incision near your navel, the doctor can look at the tubes to confirm the tubal pregnancy and then either remove the tube (salpingectomy) or remove the pregnancy from the tube (salpingostomy). Occasionally, a larger incision will be necessary to complete the operation.

Is surgery always necessary to treat a tubal pregnancy?

Most tubal pregnancies are treated surgically. If the tube has ruptured, surgery is required to stop the bleeding. Unless the doctor is certain that you have a tubal pregnancy, laparoscopy is required to confirm it. Occasionally, however, the diagnosis can be made without laparoscopy. A very early tubal pregnancy that appears to have stopped developing can be monitored without surgical intervention. If the tubal pregnancy has grown somewhat larger but there are no signs of tubal rupture, it can be treated with a medication called methotrexate, which arrests the pregnancy's development and allows the body to absorb the tissue. Methotrexate cannot be used to treat women who have liver, kidney, or peptic ulcer disease.

Can I get pregnant again after a tubal pregnancy?

Because you have two tubes and ovaries, your chances of achieving a subsequent pregnancy are good. There is approximately a 50 percent chance that you will have an intrauterine pregnancy. If you conceive, there is a 10 to 20 percent chance that you will experience another tubal pregnancy. Therefore, your doctor will want to monitor you carefully.

Sustaining two tubal pregnancies significantly diminishes the odds of future success. Only 30 percent of such women will conceive, and the odds of having another tubal pregnancy are high. In vitro fertilization (see page 93) should be considered in this situation.

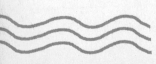

8 Endometriosis: The Great Masquerader

I was told I have endometriosis. What is that?

Endometriosis is the bane of every gynecologist's existence. You've heard the expression "a thorn in your side." Well, this is more like a spear. OK, maybe we're getting overly dramatic. Nevertheless, it can be an extremely difficult problem.

Inside the uterus is a glandular lining referred to as the endometrium. When this tissue becomes located outside of the uterus, the condition is referred to as endometriosis. There are a number of theories explaining how it gets outside. The most common hypothesis is that pieces of endometrial tissue flow back out of the fallopian tubes during the menstrual flow and become implanted on the surfaces of other organs in the pelvis, such as the uterus, ovaries, bladder, and bowel. (See the illustration on page 108.) Each month during menstrual flow, the endometrial implants bleed, causing inflammation and pain. Ultimately, scar tissue forms in affected areas. Blood from ovarian endometriosis may accumulate inside the ovary, producing a benign (noncancerous) cystic growth of the ovary, referred to as an endometrioma.

If I have painful periods, does it mean that I have endometriosis?

A common misimpression is that everyone with painful periods has endometriosis. Many women with painful periods, or dysmenorrhea, have no definable disease (see page 26). This is particularly true for those who have always had painful periods. Pain is more apt to be related to endometriosis if it is recent in origin and progressively worsening. Also, pain from endometriosis typically starts a day or two before menstrual

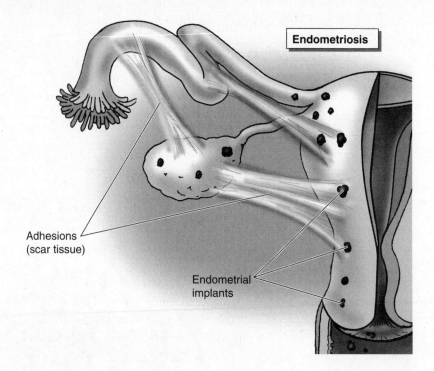

Endometriosis

Adhesions
(scar tissue)

Endometrial
implants

flow begins. Often it subsides once the flow is established. The probability of having endometriosis increases if there is a family history of the disorder.

What other symptoms characterize endometriosis?

Endometriosis can produce a multitude of different symptoms, depending on its location. That is why we call it the "great masquerader." Painful periods are the most common symptom. However, it can also cause chronic pelvic pain that is not related to the menstrual cycle. Disturbances of menstruation may also occur, and infertility is often seen in conjunction with endometriosis. Painful intercourse, occurring with deep penetration, is another fairly common symptom. Endometriosis associated with the bowel can result in painful defecation, changes in bowel function, and rectal bleeding. Urinary frequency, urinary urgency, or blood in the urine may occur if the bladder is involved.

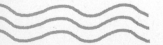

ASK YOUR GYNECOLOGIST

Well, by now you should be convinced that you have endometriosis: The fact that it can produce quite an array of symptoms is problematic. We have encountered many women throughout the years who have read or been told about symptoms of endometriosis and are now convinced that they must have it. In reality, most of them don't. Many of the same symptoms more commonly signal other medical disorders.

How is endometriosis diagnosed?

Many women have been told they have endometriosis. However, this diagnosis should be made only after laparoscopy (page 21). Your history or an exam may suggest the possibility of endometriosis, but that isn't sufficient to make a definite diagnosis.

If I have endometriosis, does that mean I can't get pregnant?

There is an increased chance of infertility with endometriosis. Adhesions (scar tissue) formed from endometriosis may obstruct the fallopian tube or encase the ovaries, thereby preventing the egg from reaching the tube. Tubal scarring can hinder the egg's movement down the tube, preventing it from reaching the uterus. Even when no adhesions are present, infertility may occur. The mechanism that causes infertility when no adhesions exist is not clearly understood.

You can find solace in knowing that most women with endometriosis and infertility will succeed in conceiving after treatment. The method of treatment depends on how severe the condition is. The American Fertility Society has developed a classification system based on the extent of the problem, the size of the endometrial implants, and the severity of adhesions. Approximately 75 percent of patients with mild endometriosis conceive after treatment. Sixty percent of those with moderate disease conceive. Patients with severe disease have a significantly lower pregnancy rate. If all else fails, in vitro fertilization may still provide an opportunity for a successful pregnancy (see page 93).

How is endometriosis treated?

There are numerous approaches. Some involve medications, usually of a hormonal nature, that reduce the endometrial implants. Surgical techniques may be used to remove the abnormal tissue and adhesions. Let's look at these approaches one at a time.

Surgery Since endometriosis is usually diagnosed by laparoscopy, surgery is often done at the time of diagnosis, using laparoscopic techniques. A telescopic instrument is placed through a tiny incision near the navel. Other small incisions are made, through which instruments are inserted to perform the surgery. Endometrial implants are destroyed, and scar tissue is removed.

Laparoscopic surgery is not always appropriate. If there is deep involvement of the bowel, ureters, or bladder, your doctor may feel that it is safer to operate through a larger incision (laparotomy). This may be more appropriate if pelvic adhesions are extensive.

Often surgical and drug treatments are combined. The most common approach is laparoscopic surgery followed by treatment with a medication called a GnRH agonist.

GnRH Agonists Because this group of medications has relatively few side effects, they are generally used as the first line of nonsurgical treatment for endometriosis. By placing the woman in a pseudomenopausal state, GnRH agonists turn off the gonadotropins that stimulate ovarian hormone production. Menstruation ceases, and the endometrial implants regress.

GnRH agonists are available in the form of injections (Lupron), as implants placed under the skin (Zoladex), or as a nasal spray (Synarel). They are effective but also very expensive, which limits their use for individuals without insurance coverage for medications. Common side effects include hot flashes, sweats, vaginal dryness, mood change, and headaches. Treatment usually takes six months. Over this time, there may be a small decrease in bone density related to the low estrogen levels. This problem seems to disappear when the treatment is finished.

Danazol A steroid closely related to male hormones, danazol (Danocrine) decreases estrogen and progesterone production, thereby eliminating the hormonal stimulation causing the growth of the endometrial implants. In addition to stopping menstruation, the drug has many side effects, including weight gain, decreased breast size, acne, oily skin, deepening of the voice, and increased facial hair. Other side effects include hot flashes, night sweats, and vaginal dryness.

After hearing this, you probably wonder who in her right mind would use danazol. But although most women will experience at least some of these problems, only about 10 percent find them sufficiently disturbing to discontinue the medication. The usual length of treatment is six months.

Oral Contraceptives Birth control pills have been used to treat endometriosis for decades, although they are less effective than GnRH agonists or danazol. Endometrial implants are less active during use of birth control pills, particularly when the pills are taken continuously without a break for menstruation.

Progesterone Progesterone alone, without estrogen, can also be used to treat endometriosis. The most common progesterone used for this purpose has been Provera, administered either orally or injected in the form of Depo-Provera. Like birth control pills, progesterone stops menstruation and renders the endometrial implants inactive. Overall, progesterone use has fewer side effects than taking combination birth control pills, although erratic bleeding is more common. Weight gain and mood change are also somewhat more likely to occur with Provera than with birth control pills. Because it delays ovulation, it is not recommended for women who have fertility problems.

Will endometriosis come back?

Unfortunately, endometriosis often reappears, even after treatment. This is extremely disconcerting after you have undergone extensive treatment to eradicate it. Symptoms may recur within months of treatment or a number of years later. Persistence is the name of the game. If one method of treatment is unsuccessful, another should be tried. You might consider consulting an infertility specialist if the endometriosis recurs, since he or she will usually have greater expertise in dealing with this disorder. If you suspect that you have endometriosis, your best bet is to start your family sooner, rather than later. If infertility has been a problem, the best window of opportunity for successful conception immediately follows treatment. Chronic pelvic pain is often associated with recurrent disease, and working with a physician who specializes in pain control can be beneficial, if one is available in your area.

Dealing with a recurrent or chronic disease is demoralizing. Seek emotional support through psychological consultation or support groups. Contact the national headquarters of the endometriosis association to find a support group in your area:

Endometriosis Association
8585 North 76th Place
Milwaukee, WI 53223
(800) 992-3636
(414) 355-2200
www.ivf.com/endoassn.html

My doctor said I'll eventually need a hysterectomy because of my endometriosis. Is that necessary?

If your primary problem is pelvic pain and childbearing is not an issue, the doctor may recommend removal of the uterus, fallopian tubes, and ovaries. Obviously, this is a very aggressive step. It is based on the rationale that endometriosis is least likely to recur if the reproductive organs are removed. Other options include conservative surgical or drug treatment. However, if you have severe symptoms that have not responded well to treatment, this more aggressive approach may be appropriate.

What happens to endometriosis after menopause?

Yeah! We finally get to say something reassuring about this disorder. Endometriosis regresses with menopause. Menopause occurs when the ovaries stop producing estrogen. Since the endometrial implants depend on estrogen, the disease lessens after menopause. However, adhesions produced by the disease will not disappear. Severe pain from the scar tissue requires surgery. If the adhesions are particularly extensive, removal of the uterus, fallopian tubes, and ovaries is a reasonable solution to the problem.

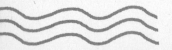

ASK YOUR GYNECOLOGIST

However, as you enter menopause, bear in mind that hormone replacement therapy must be undertaken carefully if you have a history of endometriosis. Progesterone must be given to counteract the estrogen. Cyclical regimens (those that create periodic menstrual flow) should be avoided.

9 Problems of the Uterus

What are fibroids?

Fibroids of the uterus are very common. They occur in up to 40 percent of black women and 20 percent of white women. So what is a fibroid? It's a tumor composed of smooth muscle that originates in the wall of the uterus. (See the illustration on page 115.) Fibroids vary considerably in size. They may be indiscernibly tiny or larger than a grapefruit. They can remain small throughout adulthood or grow rather quickly over a few months. Because of this variation, a gynecologist may want to examine a woman more frequently if fibroids are present, at least every six months — even if the fibroids are not causing problems.

Doctors really don't know what causes fibroids to develop. We do know that their growth accelerates in the presence of estrogen. Conditions associated with high estrogen levels, such as pregnancy, increase the growth of fibroids. Conditions with decreased estrogen levels, such as menopause, decrease their growth. There is a genetic predisposition for fibroids. If your mother or sisters have fibroids, your chance of developing them is increased.

Will my fibroids turn into cancer?

When you hear the word *tumor*, thoughts of cancer jump into your mind. Stop worrying! Fibroids are benign tumors. They can become transformed into a rare type of cancer called a sarcoma, but the incidence of this is very low — less than 1 percent. Thus fibroids should not be removed simply because of a concern that they could become malignant (cancerous).

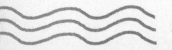

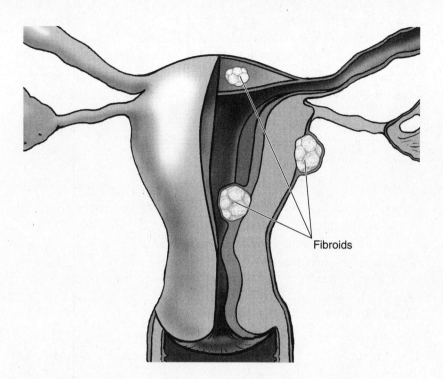

Fibroids

What problems do fibroids cause?

Actually, most fibroids never cause problems. However, numerous difficulties may be encountered. As Elizabeth Barrett Browning said, "Let me count the ways."

1. *Prolonged or heavy bleeding:* Fibroids growing into the cavity of the uterus characteristically cause heavy and prolonged periods. Occasionally, they cause bleeding between periods. The abnormal bleeding can cause anemia.

2. *Pain:* Depending on their size and position, fibroids can cause pain or pressure in the lower abdomen or back. They may also trigger pain during intercourse, particularly with deep penetration.

3. *Difficulties with urination:* Large fibroids may cause frequency and urgency of urination if they put pressure on the bladder. Occasionally,

fibroids grow in a way that obstructs the urethra, thereby creating difficulty with urinating. Very large fibroids can obstruct the ureters (the tubes carrying urine from the kidneys to the bladder). The obstruction usually causes no symptoms but nevertheless is important to address, since over time it can cause damage to the kidneys.

4. *Difficulties with bowel movements:* Pressure on the rectum can cause rectal spasms, pain with bowel movements, or difficulty with completing bowel movements.

5. *Problems with pregnancy:* Most often fibroids do not interfere with pregnancy. However, they may cause infertility or repeated miscarriages. Because of increased hormone levels during pregnancy, they tend to increase substantially in size. In doing so, a fibroid may outgrow its blood supply and degenerate, causing pain. Medication can relieve it.

When do fibroids need treatment?

Just because you have fibroids doesn't mean you have to do anything about them. Fibroids may never cause you problems. They may grow slowly or not at all. Examinations performed at six-month intervals are sufficient. However, if you are having any of the problems mentioned in the previous list, further evaluation and treatment may be necessary. If you have heavy bleeding during your period, you should see a doctor. If the bleeding is heavy enough to cause anemia, you should also consider a more aggressive approach. Remember that pelvic pain, urinary difficulties, and problems with defecation are often incorrectly attributed to fibroids and may be caused by other conditions. If you have one or more of these problems, obtain a thorough evaluation before pursuing treatment of the fibroids.

Treating fibroids prior to conception is not usually recommended. Most pregnancies progress uneventfully despite their presence. The unlikely chance that you *may* have a problem with them does not justify aggressive treatment of the fibroids. But if you experience recurrent problems that your doctor attributes to the fibroids, a more aggressive approach is indicated.

Previously, physicians recommended that exceptionally large fibroids (greater than the size of a grapefruit) be removed, even if asymptomatic. At that size, there is a greater risk that the fibroid will obstruct the ureters. It is also unlikely that your doctor will be able to check your ovaries successfully during an examination if you have very large fibroids. However, more recently this practice has been challenged. Many doctors now feel that even large fibroids do not require intervention, provided that periodic ultrasound scans are taken to evaluate the status of the ovaries and ureters.

Sometimes it is assumed that a rapidly growing fibroid needs aggressive treatment because it may be developing into a type of cancer called a sarcoma. However, even rapidly growing myomas are not typically cancerous. But if the fibroid appears to grow rapidly in menopause, a much greater problem may be present. Fibroids usually shrink during that time. Rapidly growing fibroids after menopause indicate the need for hysterectomy.

If you and your doctor do conclude that treatment of your fibroids is indicated, you must review the range of options available. They are discussed under the next two questions.

Can fibroids be treated with medications?

Until recently, medicinal therapy to treat fibroids has been largely ineffective. But the arrival of GnRH agonists (see page 110) has enhanced the management of fibroids. These medications bring about a state of false menopause. They reduce hormone levels, making the fibroids shrink, often by as much as 50 percent. That's the good news. The bad news is that the fibroids will resume their previous size when the medication is discontinued. Maximum shrinkage occurs within three months of treatment. GnRH agonists are often used before surgery to reduce the size of fibroids, thereby making the surgical procedures easier.

You may ask, "Why can't I just stay on this medication?" Unfortunately, prolonged use of GnRH agonists produces a decrease in bone density. You would also develop symptoms similar to those of menopause: hot flashes, night sweats, vaginal dryness. Researchers are searching for various ways to overcome these problems. The most common approach has been to continue treatment with the GnRH agonist while adding back a small amount of hormones to diminish the bone loss and alleviate the menopausal symptoms. Although it has achieved some success, this long-term treatment seems impractical for all but those who are close to natural menopause, when the fibroids will shrink spontaneously. In addition, GnRH agonists are extremely expensive ($250 to $300 per month), which limits prolonged therapy.

What type of surgery is used to remove fibroids?

If you and your doctor determine that surgery is necessary, fibroids can be removed through a number of techniques. Each is described here, together with a discussion of each one's potential advantages and disadvantages.

Hysterectomy The most commonly recommended treatment for fibroids in the past, hysterectomy (the removal of the entire uterus) is an option only if you no longer wish to bear children. Hysterectomy is the most aggressive approach to fibroids. Very large fibroids are removed by abdominal hysterectomy through an incision on the abdomen. Smaller fibroids are removed by vaginal hysterectomy.

Advantages

- Hysterectomy is the most thorough way of removing fibroids. More conservative methods of treatment involve the chance that more fibroids will develop and cause problems in the future, possibly requiring additional surgery.

- Removing the uterus prevents the development of other uterine problems, including endometrial and cervical cancer.

- It is easier to provide hormone replacement therapy in menopause without the uterus in place, and there are numerous benefits associated with hormone replacement in menopause (see page 169). If you have had a hysterectomy, you can take estrogen alone for hormonal replacement in menopause without worrying about an increased risk of uterine cancer or bleeding.

Disadvantages

- Hysterectomy is a major operation. Although most hysterectomies proceed without complication, chances of experiencing a com-

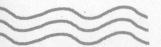

plication are greater than they would be with less invasive surgical procedures.

- Compared to laparoscopic and hysteroscopic procedures, length of stay in the hospital will be greater. The recovery period after hospitalization will also be substantially longer. If the hysterectomy can be performed vaginally, hospitalization and recuperation will be shorter than they would be for an abdominal hysterectomy.

Abdominal Myomectomy Myomectomy is an operation that removes fibroids from the uterus. An incision is made through the abdominal wall. Then incisions are made into the wall of the uterus, and the fibroids are removed. Finally, the uterus is repaired. Preserving the uterus maintains the potential for future pregnancies. However, delivery by cesarean section may be necessary after a myomectomy. Recently, some physicians have begun performing myomectomies through the laparoscope and hysteroscope.

Advantages

- The primary advantage of myomectomy is preservation of the uterus. It preserves the ability to have children.
- For some women, removal of the uterus is emotionally traumatic, and this procedure keeps it in place.
- Most physicians think that the uterus functions only in reproduction because ovaries produce hormones, not the uterus. However, other investigators say the uterus is important in pelvic support and sexual responsiveness.

Disadvantages

- If the myomectomy must be performed through a large incision on the abdomen, hospitalization and recovery are similar in duration to those of a hysterectomy.
- The time required for this surgery and the blood loss associated with it may exceed those of hysterectomy.
- Adhesions may form along the incisions made in the wall of the uterus, thereby causing infertility or pelvic pain.

- Preservation of the uterus means that other fibroids may develop in the future. If they do, the risk of requiring future surgery is 20 to 40 percent. Future fibroids may also increase chances of bleeding abnormally while taking hormone replacement during menopause.

Laparoscopic Techniques Depending on the size and location of the fibroids and the expertise of the doctor, some fibroids may be removed by laparoscopic surgery (see page 21). Only tiny incisions are made on the abdomen, and the doctor views the surgery through a telescopic instrument. Myolysis is another laparoscopic technique in which fibroids are either treated with electrical energy through needles or frozen with probes. GnRH agonists can be used to reduce the size of the fibroids first.

Advantage

- Laparoscopy requires a much shorter hospitalization and recovery period than surgery performed through larger abdominal incisions. Laparoscopy is often performed as outpatient surgery.

Disadvantages

- Advanced laparoscopic surgery requires special skills and equipment that are not universally available.
- Laparoscopic myolysis appears to be a very promising technique, but there is not yet any follow-up research on its long-term effects.

Hysteroscopic Techniques In hysteroscopy, the gynecologist introduces a telescopic instrument through the cervix into the uterine cavity. If most of the fibroid is located within the cavity, it can be removed through this procedure.

Advantage

- Hysteroscopy can be performed at an outpatient facility, and the patient recuperates quickly (there are no incisions or sutures).

Disadvantages

- It requires advanced skills and equipment that is not universally available.

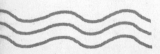

ASK YOUR GYNECOLOGIST

- It can treat only those fibroids that project well into the cavity of the uterus.

- Often the entire fibroid cannot be removed through this procedure, thereby increasing the chances of having future problems.

We should also mention a new nonsurgical treatment called embolization that looks promising. After threading a catheter into the uterine artery, physicians inject plastic particles to block the blood flow to the fibroid, which causes the fibroid to shrink. The new procedure allows patients to avoid the risks associated with surgery. Although it seems promising, more research must be done before recommending it to all women.

How can I determine which treatment for fibroids is best for me?

"But, Doctor, just tell me what I should do." Unfortunately, making this decision is not that easy. Once you and your doctor have decided that treatment is necessary, ask yourself the following questions:

1. *How close am I to menopause?* The average age of onset of menopause is 51. Your age of onset may approximate that of your mother (there seems to be a correlation). If you are close to menopause, consider managing your problem with medication as a stopgap measure. It is safe to assume that the fibroids will stop being a problem and shrink in menopause.

2. *Do I want more children?* Obviously hysterectomy is out of the question if you anticipate pregnancy in the future.

3. *How do I feel about maintaining the integrity of my reproductive organs?* If removal of your uterus will be traumatic, then all other options should be explored before hysterectomy.

4. *How do I feel about my future risk of developing cancer?* If you are very worried about cancer or there is a strong family history of uterine cancer, then hysterectomy is preferable.

5. *How do I feel about possible future problems with fibroids?* If you feel that it is important to entirely eliminate problems with fibroids in the future, hysterectomy may be your best bet.

6. *How concerned am I about the potential complications of surgery?* If you are very worried about possible complications, choose a conservative technique such as laparoscopic surgery or hysteroscopy (assuming that they are suited to your particular situation).

7. *Will I want hormone replacement therapy during menopause?* Read the section on hormone replacement therapy on page 169. If it is highly probable that you will undergo hormone replacement therapy, ask your doctor if this should influence your choice for treating the fibroids.

Can fibroids grow back?

If a fibroid is removed completely, as during a myomectomy, it will not grow back. If only a part of the fibroid is removed, there may be regrowth of the remaining portion. Fibroids that shrink during GnRH agonist treatment will return to their pretreatment size when therapy is discontinued.

If a hysterectomy is performed, you will not redevelop fibroids. However, if your uterus remains, there is a possibility that fibroids will reappear. The chance of this recurrence may be as high as 40 percent. The further you are from menopause, the more likely this will happen. However, remember that most fibroids do not cause problems. Most women who redevelop fibroids will not require treatment.

Where do polyps come from?

Uterine polyps originate from the surface lining of the uterine cavity and cervical canal. Cervical polyps can often be detected on routine examination. They tend to be small and can usually be removed in the office. Endometrial polyps are usually hidden from view inside the uterus. Often they will cause abnormal bleeding that leads to their detection.

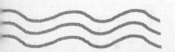

Can polyps turn into cancer?

Most endometrial and cervical polyps are benign (noncancerous). However, cancer can develop within polyps. All polyps that are removed should be sent to a pathologist, who will examine them under a microscope to rule out the presence of cancer.

How are polyps removed?

Small cervical polyps are generally removed in the office. Your doctor may administer a local anesthetic to the cervix, although most of the time this is not necessary. The polyp is attached to the cervix by a stalk. Your doctor snips the stalk with a biopsy instrument or scissors, thereby removing the polyp. You may feel a pinch when this is done, but significant pain from the procedure is uncommon.

Endometrial polyps aren't quite as easy to approach because they are located inside the uterus where they cannot be seen during examination. Most are discovered during surgery performed to determine the cause of abnormal bleeding. Any of the following conditions constitutes abnormal bleeding:

- Prolonged bleeding (duration of greater than one week)
- Exceptionally heavy bleeding
- Bleeding between periods
- Postmenopausal bleeding

In the past, the standard procedure for evaluating abnormal bleeding was a D&C (dilation and curettage). The doctor performs a D&C by dilating the cervix and placing a scraping instrument into the uterus. A sampling of the endometrium is removed and studied under a microscope. Although this procedure is very good for diagnosing endometrial cancer, it is mediocre for removing polyps.

If a pelvic scan suggests an intrauterine mass or if abnormal bleeding persists after a D&C, hysteroscopy is indicated. During hysteroscopy, the doctor inserts a telescopic instrument through the vagina and cervix into the uterine cavity and removes the polyps. This procedure can be performed at an outpatient facility. Recovery is usually quick. Varying degrees of cramping and bleeding may ensue for a short time after the procedure, but serious complications are uncommon.

My doctor said my heavy bleeding is from adenomyosis. Is that the same as endometriosis?

Patients often confuse adenomyosis and endometriosis. Endometriosis, which is discussed in chapter 8, is a condition in which endometrial tissue is located outside the uterus. Although it may be associated with abnormal bleeding, it does not usually cause heavy periods. In adenomyosis, endometrial tissue grows into the muscular wall of the uterus (the myometrium). Adenomyosis is not a cancerous condition. It most often becomes apparent in a woman's thirties or forties and manifests itself as heavy or prolonged periods.

How can the gynecologist tell if I have adenomyosis?

It is very difficult to diagnose adenomyosis. Your doctor may suspect the presence of adenomyosis if your uterus feels symmetrically enlarged and boggy; fibroids, in contrast, cause the uterus to feel irregular in shape. Heavy and crampy periods are a defining characteristic of adenomyosis. No test or procedure reliably diagnoses this condition. Certain radiologic studies or hysteroscopy (described on page 120) may suggest that this condition exists. Most often it is diagnosed by excluding other causes of heavy periods. If your periods are not improved through hormonal regulation and no polyps or fibroids have been discovered, you probably have adenomyosis.

How is adenomyosis treated?

Adenomyosis may not require any treatment. If your periods are somewhat heavy but still tolerable, you don't have to do anything. However, you should drink more fluids during your period and take an iron supplement. Over-the-counter medications such as ibuprofen (Motrin, Nuprin, Medipren) and naproxen sodium (Aleve) may help relieve cramping. Progressively heavier periods or prolonged periods require further investigation to rule out polyps, fibroids, and cancer as causes. This may include endometrial biopsy, D&C, pelvic ultrasound, and

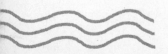

hysteroscopy. Hormonal regulation of heavy periods can be attempted, although it is not likely to succeed if you have adenomyosis.

The most successful conservative procedures used in the treatment of adenomyosis are hysteroscopic endometrial ablation and resection. With ablation, the doctor uses laser or electrocautery to destroy the endometrium. With resection, the doctor attempts to remove the endometrium with an electrocauterized loop. These procedures are performed as outpatient surgery through the hysteroscope. Recently, doctors have inserted a balloon device filled with hot liquid into the uterus to perform ablation. This technique is promising. It is easier than hysteroscopic ablation but not yet widely available. Ablation can be performed only in women who have completed their families. Endometrial sampling, either through an endometrial biopsy or D&C, must be done before the ablation, to be certain that no cancerous or precancerous condition exists within the uterus. These procedures offer an 85 to 90 percent chance of successfully eliminating or decreasing menstrual flow. The 10 to 15 percent of women whose treatments fail usually have deeply penetrating adenomyosis.

Hysterectomy is a reasonable choice for a woman with severe adenomyosis that is unresponsive to conservative approaches. Such a hysterectomy can often be performed by removing the uterus vaginally.

I'm 60 years old, and now I'm bleeding. Does that mean I have cancer?

Most women realize that it is not normal to have vaginal bleeding during menopause. If you have not bled for years and start to bleed, it is natural to feel anxious. Try to remain calm. Most postmenopausal bleeding does not indicate cancer. Often benign growths such as polyps of the cervix or endometrium will bleed (see page 122). Without estrogen replacement, the lining of the vagina and uterus becomes thin and can bleed. Another cause of bleeding after menopause is endometrial hyperplasia, a condition caused by an excess number and crowding of the endometrial glands in the lining of the uterus. Certain types of hyperplasia are considered precancerous. When discovered, hyperplasia can be reversed by administering progesterone.

It is not unusual for women on hormone replacement therapy to have bleeding (refer to chapter 13). If you are taking a hormone replacement, ask your doctor what to expect in terms of vaginal bleeding.

Certainly postmenopausal bleeding should be investigated because it may be a sign of cancer. However, don't panic. Your condition may turn out to be benign.

What is endometrial cancer?

Cancer of the inside lining of the uterine cavity, or endometrium, is referred to as endometrial cancer. The cancer begins inside the uterus and gradually extends into the myometrium, or muscular wall of the uterus. It is also not uncommon for it to extend downward into the cervix. In its more advanced stages, the cancer spreads elsewhere in the pelvis or into the vagina. If the cancer cells spread into the lymphatic drainage of the pelvis or the bloodstream, they can invade other parts of the body, particularly the lungs, liver, and bones. Fortunately, most endometrial cancers cause abnormal bleeding that prompts the doctor to investigate and discover the cancer while it is still early in development.

How did I get endometrial cancer?

Nobody completely understands why women get endometrial cancer. Estrogen stimulates endometrial growth, whereas progesterone decreases it. Conditions that produce an excess of estrogen, unbalanced by progesterone, increase the risk of getting endometrial cancer. They include the following:

- *Obesity:* Fat cells in the body convert other hormones in the body to estrogen.
- *Women with infrequent periods:* During the months that periods are missed, the ovaries are still producing estrogen. However, no progesterone is produced during those months to oppose the effects of the estrogen on your endometrium.
- *Women who have a late menopause:* The average age of onset is 51. Later onset is a risk factor.
- *Women with polycystic ovarian disease:* Women who have this disease

infrequently ovulate and develop multiple small cysts in their ovaries.

There is sometimes a genetic, or familial, predisposition to endometrial cancer. If you have a close family member who has had endometrial cancer, your risk of developing it is increased. Your risk is also greater if you have had cancer of the breast, ovary, or colon.

How is endometrial cancer diagnosed?

If you have abnormal bleeding past the age of 35 (some doctors use age 40 as a cutoff), it must be investigated. Prolonged periods, bleeding between periods, and very erratic bleeding constitute abnormal bleeding. If you are in menopause and have *any* bleeding (presuming you are not on hormone replacement), it is abnormal. Do not wait to see if it will recur. Early detection of possible cancer is the mainstay of success.

Investigation of the bleeding might include pelvic ultrasound, endometrial biopsy, D&C, or hysteroscopy (see earlier sections of this chapter). Complications from these procedures are uncommon. If you have abnormal bleeding, the need to obtain more information outweighs the risk of undergoing any of these procedures. The least invasive of the procedures is pelvic ultrasound, but it does not provide your doctor with a tissue specimen for analysis. An endometrial biopsy can be performed in the office and is an effective tool for diagnosing cancer. A D&C provides a greater amount of tissue than the endometrial biopsy but is usually performed in the operating room under anesthesia. Hysteroscopy provides the most thorough evaluation of the uterine cavity and enables your doctor to remove other benign causes of abnormal bleeding, such as fibroids and polyps. Hysteroscopy is also usually performed in the operating room under anesthesia, although some gynecologists perform it at the office.

The most important "take-home message" is that you shouldn't defer investigation of the bleeding. It may not represent cancer. However, if cancer is discovered, early diagnosis greatly increases the likelihood of a good prognosis.

Why didn't this show up on my Pap smear?

There are many misconceptions regarding the Pap smear. The most prevalent is that Pap smears screen women for all types of gynecologic malignancies. The standard Pap smear is obtained from the cervix and can detect only cervical cancer. Cancer of the endometrium begins inside the uterus and is therefore not usually detected on a Pap smear. Occasionally, malignant cells from inside the uterus "drop down" the cervical canal and are discovered on a Pap smear, but that is unusual. Abnormal bleeding must be investigated, even if a Pap smear is normal.

Do I need a hysterectomy to treat endometrial cancer?

Surgery is the mainstay of treating endometrial cancer. If it is determined that surgery would be too risky, you can be treated with radiation. If you are healthy enough to undergo surgery, your doctor will recommend an abdominal hysterectomy with removal of both fallopian tubes and both ovaries. The doctor may also want to remove lymph nodes in the pelvis or abdomen to help determine if the cancer has spread beyond the uterus. Some physicians may be willing to perform a vaginal hysterectomy or laparoscopically assisted vaginal hysterectomy (see page 125). However, most doctors who specialize in gynecologic cancer recommend an abdominal approach that allows them the best opportunity to assess the extent of your cancer.

I'm scared. What will happen if I don't do anything?

Our mouths drop open whenever we hear a patient ask this question. You will die from endometrial cancer if it is not treated. Nobody can predict how long you will live without treatment, but it is likely that you will die within a few years, and maybe sooner.

Generally this question stems from fear, not a genuine desire to avoid treatment. The word *cancer* evokes apprehension in even the bravest of individuals. You may mistakenly assume that death is inevitable if you have cancer. However, most women with endometrial cancer are diagnosed early. With appropriate treatment, the vast majority are cured. You may also be scared of surgery, particularly if you have never undergone an operation. Discuss these concerns with your

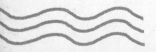

doctor. Serious complications from the surgery are uncommon. There is no doubt that the benefit from surgery far outweighs the negative but unlikely possibility of experiencing a complication.

I had a hysterectomy for endometrial cancer, and now my doctor says I need radiation therapy. Is that really necessary?

Many women will need only surgery for the treatment of endometrial cancer. However, in the following situations, additional therapy may be required:

- The cancer is assigned a high grade. High-grade cancers look particularly bizarre under the microscope. They are more likely to behave aggressively.

- The cancer penetrates deeply into the wall of the uterus. The chance of cancer cells existing outside the uterus is increased in this situation.

- The lymph nodes test positive for cancer.

- There is evidence of cancer spreading to other organs.

- The uterine cancer is a variety other than the typical endometrial cancer.

For the first three situations, radiation is recommended after surgery. It decreases the likelihood of recurring cancer. Its potential benefit must be weighed against its side effects. The radiation may cause bowel difficulties (bleeding, spasms, colitis, constipation, or diarrhea) and bladder problems (increased frequency and urgency of urination, burning, bleeding) that can persist after the treatment. Before submitting to the radiation, ask your doctor how much it will improve your chances for survival. Also consult the physician who will administer the radiation. It should be someone who specializes in radiation therapy. Inquire about the frequency and severity of side effects from this treatment. If your survival rate is increased by 15 to 20 percent by adding radiation therapy, it is probably in your best interest to proceed with it. If it is boosted by only 5 percent, it may not be warranted.

If there is evidence of cancer in distant organs (or a high probability that it will spread there), the doctor may recommend hormonal

the form of high-dose progesterone. This treatment will
cancer, but it may hold it in remission or slow its spread. If
as spread to a specific site, local radiation may be used at
casionally, chemotherapy is used to limit the spread of en-
ncer, but success with this treatment has been limited.

Can I take hormone replacement after treatment for endometrial cancer?

Most doctors will not allow you to take estrogen after being treated for
endometrial cancer. There is concern that any remaining cancer cells
will be stimulated by the estrogen and increase chances of a recurrence.
But recently, doctors have been less strict regarding that recommendation. If your cancer was detected very early, your risk of recurrence is
very low (5 percent or less). The risk must be weighed against the benefits you will receive from the estrogen (see page 169). You also must
consider the timing of your treatment. Most endometrial cancers that
recur will do so in the first five years after treatment. Recurrence after
ten years is rare. Many gynecologic oncologists now feel that hormone
replacement is permissible if your cancer was not advanced when it
was discovered and if you have been free of disease for ten years (some
use five).

How often should I see the doctor after my treatment for endometrial cancer?

Initially you will be seen frequently, possibly as often as every three to
four months. Your doctor will examine your pelvic region to feel for a
mass that could represent a recurrence. He or she also will obtain frequent Pap smears from the top of your vagina, which is one of the more
common sites for recurrence. If your cancer was more advanced,
follow-up may also include periodic pelvic or abdominal scans and chest
x-rays. The frequency of your visits can be decreased after two years,
but most physicians will recommend that you still be seen every six
months.

For more facts about endometrial cancer, contact these organizations:

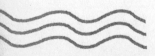

Cancer Information Service
National Cancer Institute
Building 31
Bethesda, MD 20892
(800) 422-6237
www.nci.nih.gov

The American Cancer Society
19 West 56th Street
New York, NY 10019
(800) ACS-2345
www.cancer.org

My Pap smear is abnormal. Does that mean I have cancer?

You have been taught that Pap smears are used to detect cervical cancer. Therefore, you might automatically assume that an abnormal Pap smear represents cancer. Actually, most abnormal Pap smears reflect cervical conditions that are not life threatening. Your Pap smear may become atypical because of any of the following conditions that do not indicate cancer:

- Cervicitis (infection or inflammation of the cervix)
- Irritation of the cervix from intercourse, a tampon, an IUD, or another agent
- Changes that occur as cells repair the cervix
- Changes due to inadequate estrogen levels, for example, menopause

Your doctor may want you to return to the office to be examined or to take cultures if the Pap smear suggests the presence of an infection. An infection may require specific treatment with an antibiotic or an antiviral or antifungal medication (see chapter 5). Often no infection can be identified although cervicitis is present. If the cervicitis persistently causes abnormal Pap smears, it can be treated with either cryotherapy (a freezing technique) or laser. Other changes usually reverse themselves spontaneously without specific treatment. Changes due to inadequate estrogen can be reversed with estrogen therapy.

If my Pap smear is abnormal, why did the doctor tell me to come back in three months?

It doesn't sound reasonable. After all, if the test reveals something abnormal, shouldn't you be doing something about it right away? Actually, minor abnormalities of the Pap smear often take care of themselves. If the Pap smear appears slightly atypical but doesn't show precancerous or cancerous changes, the condition is labeled benign. Most of the changes described in this section fall into this category. If there is no suggestion of infection on the smear, most doctors recommend that you wait three months, or anywhere from two to six months, and then repeat the smear. At least half of such smears will produce normal results. If the Pap smear remains atypical, further evaluation is then undertaken.

What is cervical dysplasia, and how did I get it?

Changes in cervical cells that are potentially precancerous are referred to as dysplasia (they are also called cervical intraepithelial neoplasia — CIN — or squamous intraepithelial lesion — SIL). The degree of abnormality is graded as mild, moderate, or severe. Mild dysplasia has the lowest probability of ultimately progressing to cervical cancer and sometimes spontaneously changes back to normal. Moderate and severe dysplasia have a greater likelihood of progressing to cancer.

You are at a greater risk of developing dysplasia if you began sexual activity at a young age, especially if you have had multiple sexual partners. It is more common in women with certain sexually transmitted diseases. Smokers have a greater risk than nonsmokers.

The most commonly identified cause is infection with HPV (human papillomavirus), a sexually transmitted virus that also causes genital warts (see page 74). Certain types of this virus substantially increase the chances of getting cervical dysplasia. Women who have HPV infection should have examinations and Pap smears every six months.

Cervical dysplasia doesn't always have an identifiable source. This may be disconcerting. We all want to understand the cause of a problem. However, the management of dysplasia is not affected by lack of knowledge of its cause.

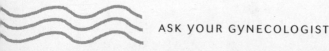

How is cervical dysplasia diagnosed?

Dysplasia is initially indicated on the Pap smear. If the Pap smear suggests dysplasia, a colposcopy is performed. This procedure takes place in the doctor's office. The doctor inserts a speculum into the vagina and examines the cervix through an optical instrument that magnifies images of the cervix. Acetic acid (vinegar) is applied to the cervix; sometimes it causes a slight burning feeling when it is applied, but usually not. The doctor will take biopsies of any suspicious-looking areas. The biopsies are sent to a laboratory for evaluation under a microscope.

How is cervical dysplasia treated?

Cervical dysplasia can be treated in various ways:

- *Observation:* Mild dysplasia may not progress and sometimes may regress. Therefore some physicians recommend that mild dysplasia be followed with frequent Pap smears (every three to four months) without further treatment unless it progresses. This is not an appropriate option for more advanced degrees of dysplasia.

- *Laser surgery:* In this procedure a high-energy beam vaporizes the dysplasia.

- *LEEP procedure:* An electrosurgical loop "scoops" the dysplasia out of the cervix. This may be followed by application of an electrosurgical ball that cauterizes the cervix.

- *Cautery:* The dysplasia is destroyed by electrosurgical techniques that apply heat.

- *Cryotherapy:* The dysplasia is treated through the application of freezing agents to the cervix.

- *Cervical conization:* If it seems possible that dysplasia or cancer may exist in the cervical canal, a cervical conization, which removes a cone of tissue from the cervix, may be recommended.

The method chosen by your doctor will depend on the severity of your dysplasia. The most common treatments are laser and LEEP procedures. If your dysplasia is severe, hysterectomy is another option if you no longer wish to have children. It is most appropriate for women who have recurring dysplasia.

Why does my doctor's treatment for dysplasia differ from the treatment received by someone I know with the same condition?

How often have we heard, "My cousin Martha has the same thing and her doctor used . . ."? Cervical abnormalities vary. Some require no treatment, whereas others are very likely to progress into cervical cancer and need intervention. Try not to compare your situation to someone else's that may not be exactly the same.

Also, two doctors may treat the same condition using different, yet equally successful, methods.

Will dysplasia come back again after treatment?

Unless a hysterectomy is performed, there is a chance that it will. Conservative treatment eradicates the dysplasia, but it doesn't remove the cervix. Dysplasia induced by HPV recurs more frequently. Also, treating the dysplasia doesn't eliminate the virus. It is important to undergo regular Pap smears (usually every six months) following treatment for dysplasia. If a Pap smear indicates recurrent dysplasia, the treatments outlined earlier are options for dealing with the condition. If childbearing is not a concern, you might consider hysterectomy, particularly if the recurrent dysplasia is severe.

If dysplasia can recur, why isn't hysterectomy always the treatment of choice?

Treating cervical dysplasia via hysterectomy is like killing an insect with a sledgehammer. Usually a less radical approach is called for. Many women will never have recurrence of dysplasia. But if you obviously are unwilling or unable to submit to regular follow-up Pap smears, hysterectomy is indicated. Hysterectomy is also reasonable if severe dysplasia persists despite repeated treatments.

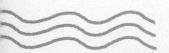

What's the difference between cervical dysplasia and cervical cancer?

Many women assume that dysplasia is an early form of cervical cancer. Many tell us that they have a family history of cervical cancer, but upon further questioning, it becomes apparent that the relative had dysplasia. *Dysplasia of the cervix is not cancer.* It is potentially, but not necessarily, precancerous. This is an important distinction. Cervical cancer mandates an aggressive approach; dysplasia does not.

How will I know if I have cervical cancer?

You probably won't know. There are no symptoms associated with early cervical cancer. That is why it is critical for you to regularly visit your doctor for Pap smears. Approximately 14,000 new cases of invasive cervical cancer are diagnosed each year. This number is dramatically lower than it was in previous decades because of Pap smear screening. Regular Pap smears will almost always detect cervical abnormalities prior to the development of invasive cervical cancer. Most commonly, cervical cancer is detected in women who have not been evaluated by a gynecologist for many years. Cervical cancer may occur at any age but is most common from age 35 to 50.

The earliest sign of cervical cancer is abnormal bleeding, particularly between periods, following intercourse, or during menopause. Don't panic! Most abnormal bleeding does not indicate cancer. Nevertheless, it needs to be evaluated. Advanced cervical cancer may cause difficulty with urination due to obstruction of the urinary tract. The tumor may also impede drainage of fluid from the legs, causing them to swell. Once again, these symptoms are much more likely to be related to other causes, but should be evaluated by a physician.

How is cervical cancer treated?

Cervical cancer is rated according to how far it has invaded. Stage I cervical cancer is confined to the cervix. Cancer that spreads beyond the cervix is categorized as stage II or stage III. By stage IV, the cancer has spread to the bowel or bladder or beyond the pelvic region.

Early cervical cancer is usually approached surgically with a radical

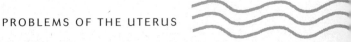

hysterectomy. The uterus and its adjacent tissue are removed. Pelvic lymph nodes and the upper part of the vagina may also be excised. If the ovaries are normal, they do not need to be removed, although this procedure is recommended for women close to menopause.

More advanced cervical cancer is treated with radiation therapy. Initially cervical cancer spreads locally, so pelvic radiation is very effective. Complications from pelvic radiation include voiding difficulties (bladder spasms, burning with urination, frequent and urgent urination) and bowel problems (rectal spasms, diarrhea). As radiation therapy has become more sophisticated, complications have become less frequent. Medications are available to help ease these symptoms, should they occur.

Cervical cancer that has spread to distant areas of the body is treated with chemotherapy. Unfortunately, successful treatment at this point is limited.

What are my chances of surviving cervical cancer?

Cervical cancer detected early has an excellent prognosis. With stage I disease, you have an 85 to 90 percent chance of surviving. Your chances decrease as the stage of the cancer increases. Cure for advanced disease that has spread to other parts of the body is very low (5 to 10 percent).

Visit your doctor regularly. A complete examination and Pap smear should be performed annually. Advanced cervical cancer is exceptionally rare in women who have regular exams.

More information on cervical cancer can be obtained from the National Cancer Institute or the American Cancer Society (see page 131).

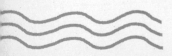

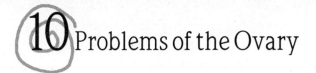10 Problems of the Ovary

I was told I have a cyst. What is that?

Any fluid-filled structure in the ovary is referred to as an ovarian cyst. Your doctor may discover an ovarian cyst when he or she examines you, or it may be detected by a radiologic scan, most often an ultrasound scan.

Sometimes the follicle containing the egg doesn't rupture at midcycle, but continues to increase in size, evolving into a follicular cyst. Sometimes the follicle does rupture, and blood collects in the follicular structure known as the corpus luteum. This is referred to as a corpus luteal, or hemorrhagic, cyst. Follicular and luteal cysts make up 90 percent of all ovarian cysts. These functional cysts clear up spontaneously. Your doctor may place you on oral contraceptives to suppress ovarian function, which some physicians believe decreases the amount of time needed to resolve the problem.

In a variation of the condition, called polycystic ovaries, unruptured follicular cysts build up within the ovaries. This abnormality is associated with infrequent ovulation that may cause infertility. Infrequent periods, obesity, and masculinizing traits such as increased facial hair may also develop.

Another type of ovarian cyst is an endometrioma, a cyst filled with old blood from endometrial tissue in the ovary.

Many types of benign (noncancerous) cystic tumors can evolve from ovarian tissue. Because most benign tumors are removed, it is not known how many of them would become cancerous if not treated.

Malignant (cancerous) tumors of the ovary may also be cystic. Fortunately, malignant tumors comprise a small minority of ovarian cysts.

Ninety-five percent of all ovarian tumors in women under age 45 are benign. The chances of a cyst being malignant increases with age, although the majority of cysts are benign even after menopause.

Why do I have pain from my ovarian cyst?

An enlarged cystic ovary may twist and turn, causing intermittent sharp pain. If the ovary is enlarged sufficiently to press on other pelvic structures, a dull, continuous pain may result. Pain may also flare up during intercourse, particularly with deep penetration. A very large cyst may be first noticed as abdominal swelling.

Occasionally a cystic ovary undergoes continuous twisting until it cuts off its blood supply. This causes profound, unrelenting pain. We're talking about the kind of pain that will bring you to the emergency room at any time, day or night. The condition is treated through surgery. Previously it required laparotomy — surgery through a large incision. Most doctors now use laparoscopic techniques (surgery using a telescopic instrument — see page 21). If it appears that the twisting process has not cut off the blood supply to the ovary, the organ can be preserved.

Rupture of an ovarian cyst also produces sharp pain. The pain then decreases in intensity but may persist as a continuous "achy" feeling in the pelvis. Diagnosis can be made if an ultrasound examination reveals "free" fluid in the pelvis from the contents of the cyst. If there is continuous bleeding from the ruptured cyst, surgery is required. However, most of the time ruptured cysts can be observed without treatment. Most ruptured cysts will resolve spontaneously. The pain usually goes away quickly, within hours or several days.

Do I need surgery if I have a cyst?

Most ovarian cysts do not require surgery. The majority will take care of themselves spontaneously over one to three months. Others will disappear after you are placed on oral contraceptives. You need surgery in the following situations:

1. Your cyst does not go away after several months, particularly if you have been placed on oral contraceptives.

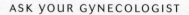

2. Your cyst is exceptionally large. If your cyst is larger than 10 centimeters, surgery may be recommended.

3. The symptoms are severe. If the pain cannot be adequately controlled, surgical intervention may be justified.

4. The cyst causes internal bleeding that does not spontaneously abate.

5. You are menopausal.

After menopause, the ovaries no longer function. If a cyst is small and is shown to have benign (noncancerous) characteristics on an ultrasound scan, the doctor may be willing to postpone surgery. A decision for postponement may be appropriate if the following criteria are met:

- The cyst must be no larger than five centimeters in size.
- The cyst must be purely fluid-filled, with no solid areas.
- The walls of the cyst must not be thickened.
- No thick walls go through the cyst (referred to as septation).
- The ultrasound scan must show no other evidence of cancer, such as free fluid in the abdomen, enlarged lymph nodes, or other tumor masses.
- You must have a normal CA-125 test. CA-125 is a blood test that screens women for ovarian cancer.
- You must be willing to undergo frequent ultrasound scans (initially every three to six months). Although a cyst may appear benign, it may grow or eventually develop into cancer.

All menopausal cysts that do not meet these criteria should be removed. Many doctors feel that all menopausal cysts should be removed if the woman is at low risk for undergoing surgery, since it is not known how many cysts will eventually become malignant. Frequent ultrasound follow-up is impractical and expensive.

What type of surgery is done for ovarian cysts?

The physician makes an incision through the abdominal wall and either removes the cyst from the ovary or extracts the entire ovary. If

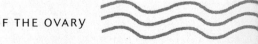

PROBLEMS OF THE OVARY

the presence of ovarian cancer is suspected, the other ovary and the uterus are also removed. Some physicians also recommend removal of the uterus and the other ovary if a woman is close to menopause. Removing them eliminates the possibility of developing future ovarian and uterine problems. This advantage must be weighed against the risk of additional surgery and the need for hormonal replacement if both ovaries are removed.

Recently, laparoscopic surgery (using a telescopic instrument) for ovarian surgery has become popular. It allows quicker recovery. Laparoscopic surgery (see page 21) for an ovarian cyst is appropriate only if the cyst appears benign.

How does the doctor know that my cyst is not cancerous?

There is no way of knowing for sure. This can be very upsetting, but it is likely that the cyst is benign, particularly for premenopausal women. If the ultrasound criteria mentioned earlier indicate that the cyst is benign and your CA-125 test is normal, then there is at least a 95 percent chance that your cyst is not cancerous. If you are premenopausal, wait to see if the cyst will resolve itself.

The doctor says I have an ovarian tumor. Does that mean I have cancer?

Words like *tumor* are tossed around cavalierly by health professionals. Without further definition, they are likely to be misinterpreted by patients. A tumor, or neoplasm, is an abnormal mass of tissue that grows more rapidly than normal. It may be noncancerous (benign) or cancerous (malignant). The word *tumor* usually denotes ovarian growths that appear to have a solid component. Fluid-filled ovarian masses that do not appear to be cysts are referred to as cystic tumors or neoplasms.

The majority of ovarian tumors are benign. The incidence of ovarian cancer increases with age, but even after menopause, more ovarian tumors are benign than malignant. Certain characteristics that can be seen on an ultrasound scan will help your doctor determine whether the tumor is likely to be cancerous. The CA-125 blood test is also helpful. However, until the tumor is removed surgically, there is no way of being sure that it is benign.

Does ovarian cancer run in families?

Most ovarian cancer occurs sporadically. It typically affects women without a family history of ovarian cancer. But in some families, women tend to develop ovarian cancer, either alone or in conjunction with breast, uterine, and colon cancers. In the general population, ovarian cancer occurs in approximately 1 out of every 70 to 80 women. It occurs more frequently in white women than black women and is most common from ages 50 to 75. The probability of developing ovarian cancer is increased for women with a history of infertility. It is also greater for those who have not had children. Childbearing and use of birth control pills decrease the likelihood of getting ovarian cancer. Tubal ligation may also have a protective effect.

If one relative in your family has had ovarian cancer, your risk is increased, but by no more than 5 percent. If multiple relatives, particularly close relatives such as your mother and sisters, have had this disease, your risk is increased substantially. This situation sometimes indicates familial ovarian cancer syndrome, a hereditary syndrome in which a defective gene increases the risk of breast and/or ovarian cancer. If you have this syndrome, your risk of developing ovarian cancer may be as high as 50 percent. Under these circumstances, most gynecologists recommend removal of the ovaries after childbearing. Even with screening, early detection of ovarian cancer is difficult. Your hormones can be replaced, but your life cannot!

Are there screening tests for ovarian cancer?

Screening tests for ovarian cancer include pelvic ultrasound and a blood test called CA-125. Routine pelvic exams will detect some ovarian cancers, although early detection by pelvic exam is uncommon. Your Pap smear does not screen you for ovarian cancer. It is valuable in detecting cervical cancer but does nothing to detect ovarian problems.

A pelvic ultrasound scan is good at revealing ovarian cysts and growths. So, why aren't we getting pelvic scans every year? First, the scans are relatively expensive, approximately $200 to $400 per scan. That's an expensive way to detect a disease that occurs in only 1.3 percent of women. Other problems limit the success of large-scale screening.

Ovarian cancer can progress rapidly. Early detection would require screening all women at least every six months. Also, ovarian cancer tends to spread to other areas in the abdomen fairly early in its course. Although screening will detect some cancers still confined to the ovary, which have a good prognosis, many will have already spread. Finally, the ultrasound scan cannot precisely determine if an ovarian growth is cancerous. Many benign ovarian cysts and tumors detected by the scan would be removed for every one that actually is malignant.

There are also problems using the CA-125 blood test. Not all ovarian cancers increase the CA-125 level. No more than 50 percent of early ovarian cancers will produce an elevated CA-125 level. On top of that, many benign conditions raise the CA-125 level. False positive elevations create anxiety and may lead to unnecessary surgical procedures. The noncancerous conditions that raise CA-125 usually occur before menopause. It is not recommended to screen premenopausal women with the CA-125 test because of this high false-positive rate. The screening is more reliable when used after menopause.

So where does this leave us? Opinions vary among gynecologists as to the value of screening for ovarian cancer. It is probably not cost-effective. However, the person who develops the cancer will find little solace in hearing that. Studies are under way to determine whether screening can actually decrease the death rate from ovarian cancer. So far, the jury is still out. If you have a family history of ovarian cancer, consider periodic screening with ultrasound and the CA-125 test. If you have an extensive family history of the disease, consult your doctor or a gynecologic oncologist as to whether you should have your ovaries removed. Also ask about genetic testing, which has become available.

What symptoms will I have if I develop ovarian cancer?

Unfortunately, you probably won't have any symptoms during the early development of the cancer, until your abdomen begins to swell. By that time, the cancer has often spread into the abdomen. The abdominal swelling is produced either by fluid in your abdomen, called ascites, or the tumor itself, which at this point may be very large. Early ovarian cancers may cause pelvic pain or painful intercourse. Occasionally the

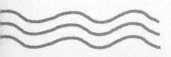

cancer will cause abnormal bleeding. Advanced ovarian cancer may create indigestion, abdominal cramps, or bloating.

Whatever you do, don't assume you have ovarian cancer if you have any of these symptoms. They all are common and are usually caused by conditions totally unrelated to cancer. On the other hand, don't ignore persistent unusual symptoms. Consult your doctor, and let him or her decide if further investigation is warranted.

If the tumor is on my ovary, why does the doctor want to perform a hysterectomy?

Ovarian cancer can spread to the uterus and may also involve the other ovary. If it is obvious that your tumor is malignant, the uterus and other ovary should be removed. If you still want to become pregnant and the cancer appears to be confined to one ovary, the uterus and opposite ovary are sometimes preserved. However, after you have completed your family, a second operation is usually recommended to have the uterus and other ovary removed. If you are near menopause (age 45 or older), your doctor may recommend removal of your uterus and other ovary, even if the tumor seems to be benign. Until the tumor is analyzed, you can't be sure that there is no cancer; and if the tumor appears benign but is found to be malignant on further evaluation, a second operation would be required. Removal of the uterus and the opposite ovary also keeps them from developing benign or malignant tumors in the future. If both ovaries are removed, hormone replacement therapy is given to prevent premature menopausal symptoms and to protect your heart and bones (see page 169).

Ovarian cancer surgery also entails removal of the omentum. The omentum is a fatty drape that lies over the intestines. It serves no worthwhile purpose and is a frequent site for metastasis (spread of cancer cells). The doctor should take biopsies throughout the abdomen and sample lymph nodes to see if the cancer has spread. He or she may be assisted by a gynecologic oncologist for this more extensive surgery. If the cancer has spread to involve the bowel, he or she may have to remove a section of the bowel to ensure the best possible prognosis after surgery.

The doctor says all the cancer was removed. Why do I have to have chemotherapy?

Even when all the visible tumor is removed, microscopic cancer cells remain in the pelvic and abdominal areas. If these are not treated, your cancer will definitely recur. In certain situations, radiation therapy will be used to treat the remaining cancer cells. However, for most types of ovarian cancer, chemotherapy is more effective. If there is no evidence that cancer has progressed beyond the ovary, chemotherapy may not be necessary. Unfortunately, only 25 percent of ovarian cancers are confined to the ovary when first diagnosed. Most women with ovarian cancer will need chemotherapy in addition to their surgery.

My uncle had chemotherapy for cancer and died anyway, so why should I take chemotherapy?

The success of chemotherapy involves many factors. Not all types of cancers respond to chemotherapy. Fortunately, most ovarian cancers respond well. Therefore, you can't compare someone else's situation to your own. Your response will depend on the following factors:

- *The extent of your cancer when it is first discovered:* If the cancer is limited, your chances of success with chemotherapy are better than if the cancer is widespread.

- *The type of ovarian cancer:* Some varieties respond better to chemotherapy than others do.

- *The grade of your cancer:* Cancers with a bizarre appearance under the microscope have a poorer prognosis.

- *The success of your surgery:* If all of the visible tumor can be removed during surgery, your chances for a positive response to chemotherapy are better than they would be if some of the tumor is left behind.

If your doctor can successfully remove all the visible cancer at the time of surgery, your chances of surviving for at least five years after chemotherapy is 50 percent. The benefit of chemotherapy in this situation clearly outweighs any risks associated with its use. If the cancer was

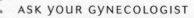

initially confined to the ovary, your chance of survival will be even higher.

The greater the extent of the cancer, the narrower the chances of survival. If the cancer cannot be fully removed at the time of surgery, your chance of surviving for five years is under 10 percent. In this situation, you must weigh the benefit of chemotherapy's potential for extending your life against the side effects you will experience. Most patients will begin chemotherapy to see if their cancer responds to it. If the tumor shrinks and the side effects from the chemotherapy are tolerable, it should be continued.

Each case of cancer is unique. Openly discuss the pros and cons of recommended treatments so that you can make an informed decision. Ask your doctor to be honest with you regarding your prognosis. If you have trouble getting information, consult a gynecologic oncologist.

Will I get sick from chemotherapy?

Side effects from chemotherapy vary, depending on what agent is used. Probably the most common side effects are nausea, vomiting, and hair loss. Medications are given to control the nausea. If your hair falls out and you're not into that Susan Powter/Sinéad O'Connor look, wear a wig until your hair grows back.

Most chemotherapeutic agents suppress bone marrow, which makes the blood cells, and thus can lead to anemia and poor blood clotting and can make you more susceptible to infections. During chemotherapy, your blood counts are monitored closely, and sometimes special drugs are administered to boost the bone marrow.

How long will I get chemotherapy?

Duration of chemotherapy ranges from 4 to 12 months. It is given in cycles, and most patients receive six to nine cycles. Each cycle lasts for three weeks. You are given the chemotherapeutic agents either as an outpatient or during a short hospitalization. The following three weeks allow your body to recover from the effects of the drugs. Throughout the course of therapy, your response to the chemotherapy will be monitored using scans (usually a CT, or "CAT" scan). The CA-125 level will also be followed if it was elevated when your cancer was initially diagnosed.

Sometimes chemotherapeutic agents are injected directly into the abdominal cavity through a catheter. Higher concentrations of the chemical reach the cancer when they are placed directly into the abdomen.

The doctor wants to look inside me again after the chemotherapy. Why?

This is referred to as a second-look operation. It is the most accurate method of assessing whether any cancer remains after your chemotherapy. CT scans can detect bulky tumors but rarely will identify tumor nodules less than two centimeters in size.

There is much controversy regarding second-look operations. It may be unwise to subject a patient to a second major operation unless the benefits are clear. Proponents of the procedure feel that it is the only reasonable method of determining if chemotherapy should be continued. However, ovarian cancer commonly recurs even when there is no evidence of persistent cancer during second-look surgery. Survival is poor in patients who continue chemotherapy when cancer is found on the second look. It is not clear that substantial benefit is to be gained from this surgery. Investigative trials are under way to try to resolve this question.

Can I be cured, or will the cancer come back?

You have a good chance of a cure if the cancer is confined to the ovary when it is discovered. Unfortunately, early ovarian cancer doesn't show symptoms. It doesn't take long for tumor cells to slough off the ovary and to implant themselves elsewhere in the pelvis and abdomen; there they evolve into tumor masses. Most women treated at this stage will eventually have a recurrence of the cancer. However, many will have prolonged periods free of disease. New chemotherapeutic agents are being discovered that offer additional hope.

If your cancer recurs, another operation and/or additional chemotherapy may be recommended. If the cancer responded well to chemo-

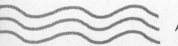

therapy previously, it may do so again, placing you in remission once more.

For more information on ovarian cancer, contact these organizations:

National Cancer Institute
Building 31
Bethesda, MD 20892
(800) 422-6237
www.nci.nih.gov

American Cancer Society
19 West 56th Street
New York, NY 10019
(800) ACS-2345
www.cancer.org

 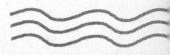

11 Problems of the Vagina and Vulva

What is that lump by my vagina?

Patients use the word *lump* to describe numerous conditions. Boils, warts, polyps, cysts, tumors, and dropped pelvic organs have all been referred to as lumps at one time or another. Normal genital structures may also be mistaken for lumps. Folds of tissue in the labia or remnants of the hymenal ring, which is located just inside the vagina, often feel lumpy but are perfectly normal.

Raised skin lesions are most likely to be warts or moles. A mole is raised and usually darker than the surrounding skin. If it increases in size or changes in shape or color, it must be removed in case it proves to be a malignant melanoma. This rule applies to any pigmented area in the vulvar region, even if it is not a raised lesion. If the mole is long-standing and doesn't seem to change in appearance, you can ignore it. Warts are usually raised skin lesions that may be more pointy than moles and usually are similar in color to the surrounding skin. Most genital warts are caused by infection with HPV virus (see page 74). Vulvar cancer may also appear as a raised area on the vulva. Consultation with a physician is imperative if you notice an unusual skin lesion: Don't assume it is a mole or wart. For best results, vulvar cancer requires early diagnosis. If your doctor finds a questionable skin lesion, he or she will biopsy it to rule out cancer.

Cysts are quite common in the genital region. If ducts in the glands located near the opening of the vagina become blocked, the gland will fill with fluid and feel like a lump. If it becomes infected, it evolves into a painful abscess and must be drained. If the gland is infected but has not developed into an abscess, your doctor will have you soak it in a

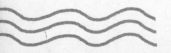

warm sitz bath (a basin that fits on your toilet seat — you can buy it in a pharmacy) or tub. He or she may also give you antibiotics. The infection will either clear up without further treatment or develop into an abscess, which is drained under local anesthesia. Vulvar cysts that are not infected do not require any treatment unless they are causing discomfort.

With the exception of vulvar skin cancer, solid tumors are less common. They include fatty tumors, nerve tissue tumors, and blood vessel tumors. These are usually benign but may warrant removal. If a solid growth has been present for many years without changing, it almost inevitably is benign. However, any new or enlarging growths should be removed.

A lump that appears to be arising from within the vagina may be a uterine or vaginal polyp. These are noncancerous growths from the lining of the vagina, cervix, or endometrium. Vaginal polyps and cervical polyps can usually be removed in the office (see page 123).

If the uterus, bladder, or rectum does not have adequate support, any one of them can descend down the vagina and appear at or beyond the vaginal opening, producing a lump. (For more information on this problem, see chapter 15.)

Why do I keep getting boils?

There are many skin glands in the pubic area. There are two types of sweat glands and oily, or sebaceous, glands. When their ducts become blocked, skin bacteria become trapped in the glands, causing pustules or boils (a big pustule). Some women have more of a tendency to develop boils in the pubic region.

When a boil occurs, you should soak it in warm water either in a sitz bath or tub. It will usually resolve by itself or will open and drain. Occasionally, a large boil must be lanced (surgically drained using a scalpel). You should keep the pubic area clean and dry to prevent recurrence. Loose-fitting cotton clothing is best. Avoid synthetic fabrics and tight slacks or underwear. Sleep in a loose nightgown or nude. Use a blow dryer (not too hot) after showering, swimming, or working out.

Sometimes boils reoccur despite preventive measures. Often one will redevelop in the same location as a previous boil and may be caused by infection of a sweat gland. Antibiotics usually do not prevent the repeated infections. Surgical removal of the infected sweat glands may be the only cure.

Why is the opening of my vagina red and painful?

If soreness is limited to the area between the inner labia at the opening of the vagina (the vestibule), you may have an obscure condition called vulvar vestibulitis. You may have one or more painful areas that are tender to touch within the vestibule. Often intercourse is exquisitely painful, precluding penetration of the vagina. Vestibulitis is very difficult to diagnose. Skin disorders, infections, allergic and irritant reactions, inflammation associated with estrogen deficiency, and trauma from activities such as bicycle and horseback riding should be excluded before the condition is diagnosed as vestibulitis.

The treatment is even more perplexing than diagnosis. Various creams and ointments (anesthetic or anti-inflammatory) may provide some relief and are usually tried first. Laser treatments have been used with varying degrees of success; however, a bulletin from the American College of Obstetrics and Gynecology does not recommend it for this condition. Ultimately, surgery may be required to remove the painful vestibular tissue. If your gynecologist has had limited exposure to this condition, consult a vulvar specialist. No, we're not kidding. They really do exist.

I constantly have burning in my vulva, but my doctor says there is nothing wrong. What can I do?

Vulvodynia is a general term that denotes vulvar pain. Burning sensations are present without obvious cause. The condition may result from injury or irritation of the nerves that supply sensation to the vulva. Other scientists postulate that high levels of an acidic salt in the urine or spasms in the pelvic muscles cause this condition. There are reports of improvement in the condition among women trained to exercise these muscles (see page 183). Hypersensitivity to yeast, allergic reactions, and skin diseases must be excluded before the diagnosis is made. Vulvar vestibulitis may be considered a kind of vulvodynia (see the previous question). Another type of vulvodynia, called pudendal neuralgia,

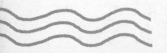

is a chronic nerve-pain syndrome, which can be treated with antidepressants or medications used to treat seizures.

Chronic vulvar pain can be very demoralizing. Doctors may tell you
that there is nothing abnormal, implying that it is "all in your head."
You know that there is something wrong but cannot get help. First you
must locate a doctor who acknowledges the existence of your problem.
If he or she is not well versed in the peculiarities of vulvodynia, ask for a
referral to someone who is. Unfortunately, it may be difficult to find an
effective treatment. For more information on vulvodynia and support
groups, contact these organizations:

The National Vulvodynia Association
P.O. Box 19288
Sarasota, FL 34726-2288
(941) 927-8503
www.ivf.com/nvabackg.html

The Vulvar Pain Foundation
Post Office Drawer 177
Graham, NC 27253
(910) 226-0704

The doctor wants to do a biopsy of the skin on my vulva. Does that mean I have cancer?

Your gynecologist should biopsy any skin abnormality involving the
vulva. It is very difficult to accurately assess vulvar skin changes based
on their appearance. Using local anesthesia in the office, your doctor
can remove a small piece of skin for microscopic analysis. Most changes
are not cancerous. Inflamed skin is often due to contact dermatitis or
vulvar infection. If this is obvious from the skin's appearance, treatment
can be done without a biopsy.

Precancerous changes in the skin of the vulva are referred to as
VIN, vulvar intraepithelial neoplasia. The degree of change is graded as
mild, moderate, or severe. In its most severe form, it is referred to as
carcinoma in situ. A small proportion of VIN cases progress to vulvar
cancer. Progression occurs slowly. If you or your doctor regularly examines the vulva, there is a good chance of early detection.

VIN can be removed with surgery or laser treatments. When the disease is widespread, the skin is removed and a skin graft is then used to re-cover the vulva.

You should strive to learn self-examination. Wash your hands thoroughly, and get into a comfortable position that will enable you to view the vulvar region with a hand mirror. You don't have to be a contortionist, although experimentation may be required. Move the mirror as necessary to look at the inner and outer labia, clitoris, vaginal and urethral openings, perineum, and perianal region (see the illustration on page 11). Any skin lesions, such as ulcerations, warts, and moles, should be noted. Pay attention to their size, shape, and color, and bring them to the attention of your doctor. Also note any change in the texture and color of the skin. Special attention should be given to pigmented areas. Don't have an anxiety attack if you discover something unusual. Remember: Most changes are not malignant!

Your doctor may also want to examine the vulva under magnification. Various dyes or acetic acid may be used to enhance the visibility of subtle areas of VIN or cancer. They direct your doctor to tissue that should be biopsied.

How is vulvar cancer treated?

Vulvar cancer develops within the skin covering the labia, clitoris, vestibule, perineum, and perianal areas. Most often it evolves from VIN (see the previous question). Vulvar cancer may emerge as a growth on the vulva but often appears as a change in skin color or texture. Alert your doctor to any change in the appearance of skin in the vulvar region.

When invasive cancer is detected during biopsy, more advanced surgery is necessary. The surgery removes the cancerous tissue, along with some of the surrounding normal tissue. In advanced cases, the entire vulva is removed (radical vulvectomy). Usually, lymph nodes near the groin are also removed. If the lymph nodes are cancerous, radiation therapy will be needed to prevent recurrence or spread of the cancer.

Early detection of vulvar cancer has an excellent prognosis. Ninety percent of patients with small lesions (defined as less than two centime-

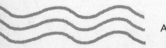

ters in size) and no enlargement of lymph nodes will survive. This confirms the benefit of self-examination mentioned earlier.

Another form of cancer seen on the vulva is Paget's disease, which is a type of skin cancer. Symptoms are persistent soreness and itching. The skin may appear thick and whitened or have well-demarcated red patches.

Malignant melanoma is a skin cancer that arises in pigmented areas of skin. Many women have a pigmented area or mole present on the vulvar skin. Any change in the size, shape, or color of such an area needs prompt medical attention. Melanomas are treated with radical vulvectomy and removal of lymph nodes.

Can you get vaginal cancer?

Yes, but it is uncommon. The doctor examines the vagina during a pelvic examination. If there is an abnormality, he or she will obtain a Pap smear or biopsy. Precancerous changes are treated conservatively with local surgery or laser vaporization. Treatment of invasive cancer is similar to that used for cervical cancer if it is located in the upper vagina and similar to the treatment for vulvar cancer if it is found in the lower vagina.

If your uterus and ovaries have been removed, you should still see a gynecologist to screen you for vaginal and vulvar cancer. You should get a Pap smear every three to five years after hysterectomy. If the hysterectomy was performed to treat cervical or endometrial cancer, you'll need to have a Pap smear annually or even more frequently if the cancer occurred recently.

More information on vulvar or vaginal cancer may be obtained from the National Cancer Institute or the American Cancer Society (see page 147).

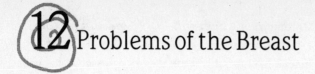

Why do my breasts hurt?

This may be the most frequently raised question in this entire book! Most women will ask it at one time or another. Besides the discomfort, there is the concern that something must be wrong if the breasts hurt. However, pain and tenderness in the breasts are quite common and only rarely reflect an ominous situation.

The exact cause of breast tenderness is unclear, although it appears to result primarily from an exaggerated response of breast tissue to the female hormones estrogen and progesterone. Normal breast tissue is composed of glands, ducts, fat, and fibrous tissue. The glands may become cystic (enlarged and full of fluid), and nodules of fibrous tissue can form within the breast. When these changes are very pronounced, doctors refer to the condition as fibrocystic breast "disease" (FBD). Doctors recognize many different variations of FBD, depending on microscopic appearance.

You will experience FBD as pain and tenderness associated with an increase in lumpiness. The condition usually worsens premenstrually, which is why you should examine your breasts and have mammograms early in your menstrual cycle. The changes may be localized to a specific area within your breast or involve the entire breast. Fibrocystic changes may be present in one or both breasts.

Many approaches have been used to reduce breast tenderness. Reducing nicotine (another reason to stop smoking) and caffeine (coffee, tea, cola, chocolate) is often recommended by physicians. Supplemental vitamin E (400 to 800 international units per day) is also frequently given. Most studies of caffeine reduction and supplemental

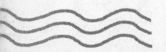

vitamin E have concluded that they are of little or no benefit. However, anecdotal reports (based on the personal experience of patients and physicians) suggest that some women find these measures useful. Over-the-counter analgesics (Tylenol, Motrin) may provide some relief. Studies indicate that FBD can be alleviated with the use of oral contraceptives. Other hormonal agents used to treat breast tenderness include these:

- Danazol (see page 110)
- Bromocriptine (also used to suppress lactation)
- Tamoxifen (an anti-estrogen; see page 163)

Each of these agents has side effects that limit its usefulness, but they should be considered if your discomfort is severe.

Does FBD increase the risk of breast cancer? This question has been debated for decades without resolution. Some studies have demonstrated a two- to fourfold increase in the risk of developing breast cancer for women with FBD. Other investigators feel that the relationship, if any, is tenuous. Certain types of FBD may increase risk, whereas others do not. Clearly, fibrocystic breasts are more difficult to examine and may make it difficult to obtain clear images through mammography.

Try to examine your breasts even if you can't interpret what you are feeling. Develop a mental image of your breasts. Describe to yourself the position and size of nodules and ridges. Thus you can create a mental "topographical map" of your breasts. After several monthly self-examinations, you will have a good feel for the contours and texture of your breasts. If there is a change in them, you will be as likely to detect it as your doctor (see page 161 for more information on self-examination).

Are breast implants dangerous?

Breast implants are used in breast augmentation (enlargement) surgery as well as reconstructive surgery following mastectomy (removal of all or part of the breast). Implants have an outer shell of silicone, similar in texture to a thick plastic freezer bag. The shell is filled with either silicone gel or saline solution (salt water). The implant is placed under the breast tissue or chest wall muscles through a small incision.

Breast implants containing silicone gel have been used for more than 20 years. There have not been extensive studies in women to establish their safety. It has become evident that the silicone from these implants "bleeds" or "sweats" through the outer shell, causing a reaction in the tissue around the implant. There is concern that silicone may also travel to other areas in the body and cause problems. Silicone breast implants have been reported to induce autoimmune diseases such as systemic lupus and rheumatoid arthritis. Because of these concerns, the FDA placed limitations on the use of silicone gel implants in 1992. Since then, several studies have compared women with and without silicone gel implants. The results do not indicate a greater incidence of autoimmune disease in women with implants. It will be several more years before results from controlled clinical trials are available to conclusively answer the safety concerns regarding silicone gel implants. In the meantime, the FDA does *not* recommend that women remove the implants if they are not having problems.

Implants filled with saline solution are being used for augmentation and breast reconstruction in place of silicone gel implants. More work needs to be done to establish the safety of these as well. Saline is nontoxic to the body, so it is unlikely that saline implants pose a substantial health risk.

The most common complication of breast augmentation occurs when the body forms a hard fibrous capsule around the implant. Called capsular contracture, the condition produces a firm breast that has lost its soft, natural texture. The breast may also become painful. Fortunately, improved implants and surgical techniques have decreased the frequency of this complication. When the problem is severe, a second operation may be required to correct the problem or remove the implant. Occasionally, decreased nipple sensitivity will occur after breast augmentation. A breast implant may also rupture or deflate. When this happens, it must be replaced to maintain breast symmetry.

Recently breast implants filled with soybean oil have been developed. Clinical trials are under way, and initial results are promising. The implants are translucent, permitting a clear mammographic view of the breast. Soybean oil is readily metabolized by the body in the event that the implant leaks or ruptures. More testing is required before the FDA grants approval of soybean oil implants, but they appear to be better and safer than other implants.

Can anything be done if my breasts are too large?

Exceptionally large breasts create numerous problems. They often produce a sense of heaviness and pain, particularly before a menstrual period. Large breasts cause shoulder, neck, and upper-back strain, resulting in pain in those regions. Chronic skin irritation may develop in the folds under the breasts.

Breast reduction is a surgical procedure that reduces the volume of tissue. It can significantly improve the comfort and quality of life in women with abnormally large breasts.

However, there are drawbacks. (Why does there always have to be a catch?) Breast reduction involves rather extensive incisions. Scar formation along these incision lines can be unsightly. Lactation and breast-feeding may not be possible following this surgery. There may also be decreased sensitivity of the nipples. Nevertheless, most women who undergo breast reduction surgery are pleased. The relief obtained seems to outweigh the shortcomings of this procedure.

I have a tender area in my breast. Does this mean I have cancer?

A tender area within the breast is usually a cyst. This diagnosis can be made by ultrasound or by drawing fluid out of it. Breast cancer is not typically associated with tenderness. It is more apt to appear as a painless, hard lump. Other causes of tenderness include injury to the breast, inflammation caused by an infection, superficial phlebitis (inflammation of a vein), and inflammatory breast cancers. Fibrocystic breasts do not appear inflamed (no redness, heat, or swelling) and are not associated with fever. If you develop localized tenderness associated with either fever or inflammation, contact your doctor.

Why does the doctor want to draw fluid out of the lump in my breast?

Most breast lumps are benign cysts. Your doctor may attempt to take out some fluid to confirm the lump is cystic. Once that is done, the lump should disappear. Sometimes the fluid is sent to a laboratory for analysis. Most solid lumps should be biopsied. Don't assume that the lump is cancerous if your doctor cannot take fluid from it. The lump may be composed of fibrocystic tissue. It may also be a benign solid tumor.

What does it mean if I have a discharge from my nipple?

Nipple discharge is fairly common and usually does not indicate a severe problem. Almost half of women in their reproductive years can express a few drops of liquid from their breasts. In fact, squeezing the nipple during self-exams is no longer encouraged by the American Cancer Society, although you should still look for spontaneous discharge and report it to your physician.

A milky discharge from the nipple is normal during pregnancy. It is also common up to one year after nursing is stopped. It is not common at other times. Most of the time it is white or clear, although it may also appear yellow or green. Yellow or green discharge may signal a disease of the breast.

Discharge from the nipple may be caused by the following factors:

- Birth control pills
- Certain medications (ask your doctor to check the *Physician's Drug Reference* to see if it is listed as a side effect)
- Prolonged and intense suckling
- Conditions that stimulate the nerves in the chest wall, such as shingles, chest surgery, and lesions in the upper spinal cord
- Hypothyroidism (deficient thyroid hormone indirectly stimulates lactation)
- Central nervous system injuries or tumors that affect the pituitary

gland, which is located at the base of the brain and controls the secretion of many important hormones

- Pituitary tumors

If you have a discharge, your doctor will order tests to check the level of prolactin, the hormone responsible for the production of breast milk. He or she may also check your thyroid. If prolactin is elevated, the doctor may order a scan to rule out a pituitary tumor. A pituitary tumor can usually be treated with a medication that shrinks it. Occasionally, surgery will be recommended.

Nipple discharge may also contain pus or appear watery, yellow, multicolored, or bloody. Discharge containing pus is usually caused by a bacterial infection and is accompanied by pain, tenderness, redness, and swelling. This infection (called mastitis) is most common after pregnancy, especially during nursing. Bloody discharge is of greater concern since it may be a sign of cancer. But not all bloody discharges are caused by cancer. In fact, the most likely culprit is a benign growth, known as an intraductal papilloma, which is located within one of the breast ducts, usually near the nipple. Discharges may also be a sign of a breast disease called ductal ectasia. Fibrocystic breast disease can cause nipple discharge.

Further evaluation is necessary if you have a nipple discharge, particularly if it is bloody. Your doctor will examine your breasts for lumps and obtain a mammogram or other radiologic tests. Analysis of the fluid will usually be performed. The treatment of nipple discharge varies according to the cause. Mastitis is treated with antibiotics. Ductal ectasia is treated by bed rest, ice packs, and anti-inflammatory drugs. Surgical excision may be required if the condition persists or if a mass develops. Papillomas are removed through minor outpatient surgery. Areas that look suspicious are biopsied to see if they are cancerous.

Is there anything I can do to prevent breast cancer?

There are many risk factors involved in breast cancer. Most of these are beyond your control. Women with a strong family history of breast cancer are at greater risk. So are women who began menstruating early or who enter menopause late. Women who delay childbearing are also more susceptible.

Nutritional factors are within your control, however. Most studies show an increased risk of breast cancer with obesity (particularly if the weight is concentrated at the waist). It also increases with alcohol consumption (more than three drinks per week). Maintaining a healthy diet that is low in fat and alcohol may reduce the risk of developing breast cancer.

The role of estrogen and progesterone in the development of breast cancer has not been firmly established, and controversy characterizes ongoing research and debate. Birth control pills probably do not increase the overall risk of developing breast cancer. The role of hormone replacement therapy in breast cancer remains more controversial. For a discussion of this topic, see page 177.

Is my risk of developing breast cancer increased if my mother had it?

Family history is definitely important in assessing your risk of getting breast cancer. If you have a close relative, such as a mother or sister, who develops breast cancer, your risk is doubled. This is particularly true if the cancer appeared before menopause. If multiple female members of your family have been diagnosed with either breast or ovarian cancer, your risk may be as much as 50 percent or higher. The inherited tendency can be transmitted through the maternal or paternal side of your family, through an abnormal gene. Women may be genetically screened for this abnormality. If multiple female members of your family have had ovarian or breast cancer, you should consult a geneticist to assess your risk.

What can you do if it is determined that your risk is very high? You should do self-exams monthly and have breast exams by a physician every six months. Get an annual mammogram starting at an early age (determined by the age at which breast cancer developed in your relatives). Removal of both breasts has been suggested as a proactive measure. It *reduces* the risk of breast cancer but does not eliminate it entirely because surgery may leave behind breast tissue along the chest wall. Tamoxifen, which is currently used in the treatment of breast cancer (see

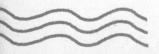

ASK YOUR GYNECOLOGIST

page 163), has also been proposed for the prevention of breast cancer. Clinical trials are under way to evaluate this option.

How can I tell if I have breast cancer?

There are no symptoms associated with the early stages of breast cancer. Early detection is possible only through breast exams, physician exams, and screening mammograms. The most common finding is a painless, hard lump. If you or your physician detects a lump, it must be investigated, even if your mammogram is normal. Other signs include the following:

- *Discharge from your nipple, particularly if it is bloody:* However, remember that most bloody discharges are caused by intraductal papillomas, which are not cancerous. Don't panic!

- *Nipple inversion:* If your nipples normally point outward, nipple inversion (nipples pulled inward) is considered ominous. This does not apply to women with chronically inverted nipples.

- *Certain skin changes:* Sometimes the skin overlying a breast cancer develops the texture of an orange peel. Dimpling of the skin may be caused by an underlying cancer. Finally, inflammatory cancers may cause the breast to appear red and swollen, although some noncancerous conditions also present with inflammation.

- *A lump in your armpit:* This may reflect an enlarged lymph node caused by breast cancer.

Perform monthly breast examinations. Premenopausal women should do the exam early in the cycle to avoid the increased lumpiness and tenderness that come just before menstruation. Lie on your back, and place one arm over your head. With your other arm, reach over and examine your breast. Move your fingers in a pattern such as concentric circles to ensure that no area of the breast is missed. Include the armpits in your examination. Keep your fingers flat and the pressure light to maximize your ability to sense changes in the breast tissue. Perform the same procedure on the opposite breast. Some women find the examination easier in the shower or bath when skin is wet and slippery. Ideally, you should perform the exam in both upright and lying-down positions.

Next, look at your breasts. Stand in front of a mirror with your arms behind your head. Look for any changes in the size or shape of your breasts. Identify any change in the skin texture or color, as well as any dimpling of the skin. Make sure there is no inversion of the nipples.

Remember that the primary responsibility for your health rests with you, not your doctor. Bring any abnormalities to your doctor's attention. The survival rate with early breast cancer detection is excellent. Breast exams, coupled with physician exams and mammography, provide you with an excellent chance for early detection.

When is a breast biopsy necessary?

Most solid lumps should be biopsied or removed. Scattered calcium deposits in breast tissue are common and usually do not warrant biopsy. However, suspicious clusters of calcifications should be biopsied. If a lump is cystic (see page 154), biopsy is not necessary.

Biopsies can be performed in several different ways. The doctor may remove the entire lump, which is called an excisional biopsy. However, he or she may choose to pass a needle through the lump to collect cells or pieces of tissue that are then analyzed. If the mass cannot be felt, a radiologist will use one of a variety of techniques to help the doctor locate and biopsy the area in question.

Do I need to have my entire breast removed if there is cancer?

A radical mastectomy removes all the breast tissue, along with the overlying skin and underlying muscles. The lymph nodes under the armpit are also removed. Radical mastectomy remained the treatment of choice until the 1970s, when earlier diagnosis of breast cancer made less radical surgery possible. This development led to a preference for the modified radical mastectomy, which preserves the pectoralis muscle (the large muscle in the front of the chest, under the breast). More recently, studies have indicated that the breast can often be saved. If the breast cancer is discovered early, the cancer can often be removed while preserving the rest of the breast. This operation is called a lumpectomy. A lumpectomy must be followed by radiation therapy and removal of

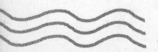

the lymph nodes under the armpit to determine whether the cancer has spread.

Surgeons do not always agree on what constitutes the best surgical approach to breast cancer. Breast-conserving surgery is not best in all cases. You must discuss this with your doctor to see if it is a reasonable choice. This is one area in which a second opinion may be very useful.

Why do I need radiation therapy after a lumpectomy?

Cancer cells will migrate from the main cancerous lump. The spread of these cells can cause the cancer to recur. The cells can also enter the bloodstream or lymphatic system, allowing the cancer to spread to other parts of the body. Radiation is given for five to seven weeks to eradicate cancer cells remaining in the breast after lumpectomy. It may cause some fatigue over the course of treatment. Other side effects include skin changes (dryness, redness, or tanning), swelling, and muscle stiffness. Most effects from the radiation disappear within a few weeks after the completion of treatment, although swelling may persist longer. Severe complications from radiation therapy are rare.

When is chemotherapy necessary?

Some women with breast cancer in the earliest stages can be treated with surgery alone or lumpectomy with radiation. Many women, however, will receive chemotherapy after surgery. Breast cancer in premenopausal women can spread quickly if not treated aggressively, so most premenopausal women will receive chemotherapy as part of their treatment.

Occasionally, chemotherapy is started before surgery. This step is usually taken when the cancerous lump is large, and it is suspected that cancer cells have already spread beyond the breast. Preoperative chemotherapy may shrink the size of the lump, thereby allowing more conservative surgery.

Chemotherapy is usually given for four to six months. (For a discussion of common side effects, see page 145.)

What is hormonal therapy?

Breast cancer is tested to see if there are estrogen receptors on the surface of the cancer cells. If they are present, an anti-estrogen called tamoxifen (Nolvadex) will be prescribed to decrease the risk of recurrence. Tamoxifen is usually taken for five years. Side effects are usually mild. The most common adverse reactions include hot flashes, nausea and vomiting, menstrual irregularities (in premenopausal women), vaginal discharge, and skin rash.

Tamoxifen does have risks associated with its use. Some studies indicate a small increased risk of blood clots in the veins, but this is difficult to evaluate. It has become evident that endometrial polyps and endometrial cancer (see page 126) are more likely to develop during treatment with tamoxifen. This may seem to be trading one cancer for another! Fortunately, it is relatively easy to monitor the condition of the endometrium. Ultrasound studies and endometrial biopsies can detect problems, and one or both of these studies should be performed yearly during treatment with tamoxifen. If endometrial cancer develops, it will be diagnosed early when it is completely curable.

Like estrogen, tamoxifen protects woman against osteoporosis and decreases the risk of getting a heart attack.

I hear that the breast can be reconstructed. Is that true?

Breast reconstruction is a major advance in the rehabilitation of patients undergoing mastectomy. Loss of the breast can be psychologically devastating, and 30 to 40 percent of women report a loss of sexual desire or reduction in arousal following mastectomy, despite the fact that most relationships remain intact and, on occasion, even are strengthened. Breast reconstruction can restore a woman's sense of femininity and sexuality.

Traditionally, breast reconstruction was delayed until it was determined that there was little risk of recurrence of the cancer. Now breast reconstruction can often be performed immediately following the mastectomy. Not all physicians agree that immediate reconstruction is best, believing that risk of surgical infection is increased and recuperation delayed. Delayed reconstruction also may result in a cosmetically superior breast. Not every woman is a candidate for immediate reconstruction, but it should certainly be discussed with a physician before mastectomy.

Not all women perceive mastectomy as disfiguring. Some feel comfortable wearing an external prosthesis. This choice has the advantage of decreasing the amount of surgery. A woman can always change her mind and undergo breast reconstruction later.

If you have breast cancer and would like additional information or support, contact the following resources:

Reach to Recovery
American Cancer Society
19 West 56th Street
New York, NY 10019
(212) 586-8700
www.cancer.org

Y-Me National Organization for Breast Cancer Information and
    Support
212 West Van Buren
Chicago, IL 60607
(312) 986-8228 (24 hours)
(800) 221-2141
www.Y-me.org

National Cancer Institute
Building 31
Bethesda, MD 20892
(800) 4-CANCER
www.nci.nih.gov

13 Menopause and Hormone Replacement: The Great Debate

When will I reach menopause?

As age 40 rolls by, thoughts turn to menopause. Half of you are looking forward to menopause and "getting rid of that darn period." The rest of you are dreading its arrival. The majority of women will cease menstruation between ages 48 and 55; the average age of onset of menopause is 52. However, it is not rare for a woman to stop menstruating as early as age 40 or to persist into her late fifties. There does appear to be a correlation with the age at which a woman's mother entered menopause and the age at which she will reach it herself. Skipped periods and hot flashes or night sweats signal the approach of menopause. These first signs indicate that a woman is perimenopausal (close to menopause).

What is a hot flash?

You want the windows open. He wants them shut. What the heck is going on here? You may be experiencing hot flashes. Also referred to as hot flushes, hot flashes are sudden, warm feelings throughout the head, neck, and chest area. They may be quite dramatic. Often they appear with perspiration, particularly at night. They may also be accompanied by insomnia, dizziness, or palpitations. A general sense of warmth or intolerance to heat is not considered a hot flash. Hot flashes are directly related to a reduction in estrogen production. They are usually most prominent after menstruation has ceased completely but may begin while you are still intermittently getting periods.

The most effective treatment for hot flashes is estrogen replacement therapy. Progesterone may provide some relief when given alone but is not as good as estrogen in providing relief.

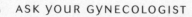

Why is sex painful since I stopped getting periods?

You've stopped getting periods. Terrific! Now you don't have to worry about getting pregnant. This should put a shot of adrenaline into the ol' sex life. But wait, something isn't right. Intercourse is painful. You have vaginal dryness and burning. What's happening? You probably have vaginal atrophy.

Estrogen sustains the lining of the vagina. Without estrogen, the lining thins and loses its elasticity. The normal moisture of the vagina is reduced, causing dryness and irritation. These factors make intercourse painful. The vagina may even burn or itch without sexual activity, a condition that is called atrophic vaginitis. The lining of the bladder also atrophies and may cause symptoms of urinary burning or urgency.

Atrophic vaginitis is corrected with estrogen replacement therapy. Within several months of beginning estrogen replacement, the vagina will regain its normal elasticity and lubrication. Even small amounts of estrogen cream administered vaginally once or twice weekly can reverse the changes. Nonhormonal moisturizing products (Gyne-moistren, Replens) are also available to help those experiencing vaginal dryness. They are particularly useful for women who should not have estrogen replacement. Products are also available that enhance lubrication during intercourse (Lubrin, Vagisil Intimate Moisturizer), although you may find that ordinary K-Y jelly works just as well. These nonhormonal preparations are available over the counter in the feminine hygiene section of your pharmacy or supermarket.

I don't seem to have any sex drive. Is that because of menopause?

"I used to have a great sex drive. Now I'd just as soon see him go out with his buddies. What's wrong?"

Decreased libido, or sex drive, is a frequent occurrence in menopause. You may also experience diminished sensitivity in your nipples and clitoris. Decreased arousability can then reduce your capacity for orgasm. If decreased libido is a significant problem for you in menopause, your doctor can begin estrogen replacement therapy. If this does not correct the problem, a small amount of testosterone can be added to the hormone replacement, either separately or combined with your estrogen. Estratest combines both hormones in one tablet.

Decreased libido often arises from factors unrelated to hormone production (see pages 59–60).

I feel depressed. Does menopause cause that?

Menopause is not associated with depression for most women. However, decline in the production of ovarian hormones may induce mood disturbances. In menopause, women may experience depressed mood, fatigue, irritability, anxiety, and sleep disturbances. It is not known whether these are directly attributable to the decrease in estrogen. Women at high risk for depression during menopause include those with a past history of depression or severe PMS and those with a family history of depression.

There may be other nonhormonal reasons for depression. Menopause occurs during midlife, a time of transition. Many women who have previously invested time and energy into raising children must redefine their role and explore other avenues for fulfillment. Midlife is often accompanied by other stresses. You may have to care for infirm parents. You or your partner may have health problems. Friends may be lost through illness or relocation. Coping with these and other midlife challenges may be difficult and lead to mood disturbances.

You don't have to know whether your mood changes are directly attributable to declining ovarian function. Unless there is a medical reason not to, your doctor can begin estrogen replacement therapy. Estrogen enhances mood in many women during menopause. Adding testosterone to the hormone replacement regimen may elevate mood better than estrogen alone. If you magically turn into a new person, the mood changes were probably related to the decrease in your hormones. If the problem continues or is particularly severe, you should consider consulting a psychologist or psychiatrist.

As you approach menopause, consider all the positives. The departure of your children creates more time for you to explore new activities and hobbies. It may give you the opportunity to reenter the workforce or devote more time to your current job. Perhaps you can finally travel to those places you couldn't go to while the children were at home. You and your husband may have the chance to spend more time alone, thereby strengthening your relationship. Your sex life may flourish now that you are freed from concerns about unplanned pregnancy. You have acquired wisdom and insight throughout your life that enable you to tackle challenges that weren't approachable in your youth. Climb every mountain. . . . Ford every stream. . . .

Why do I hear so much about hormones?

Estrogen relieves menopausal symptoms. But a couple of decades ago, when it became apparent that estrogen also increases the risk of endometrial cancer, hormone replacement came to a screeching halt. Since that time, safer ways of giving estrogen have been found, so women can now enjoy the benefits with less risk. Estrogen replacement has at least two major health benefits: protection of the bones and protection of the heart.

One out of five women is disabled by the age of 70 by osteoporosis, or thinning of the bones. One and a half million fractures related to osteoporosis occur in this country every year. Of those, approximately 300,000 are hip fractures, and 15 to 20 percent of the women who sustain them die from complications of hip fracture. Of those that survive, only about one half are able to walk unassisted, and 25 percent are restricted to long-term care facilities. The spinal column and forearm are also common sites for fractures related to osteoporosis.

Your aunt Millie, who was stooped over, didn't have poor posture. The vertebrae in her spinal column were crumbling. Estrogen replacement helps prevent osteoporosis in menopause, dramatically reduces the rate of bone loss, and decreases the risk of getting fractures and spinal deformity such as the curvature of the upper back referred to as "dowager's hump."

Protection of the heart against coronary artery disease is the other major health benefit gained from estrogen replacement therapy. As a group, women on estrogen have a 40 percent lower chance of getting a heart attack compared to women not on estrogen replacement. One out of every two women will die from heart disease. The risk of developing heart disease usually far outweighs the risk of developing all cancers combined. Estrogen causes levels of good cholesterol (HDL) to rise, while bad cholesterol (LDL) decreases. Estrogen also appears to directly affect the coronary arteries in the heart. It is not clear if it offers protection against stroke. The data seem to indicate that risk of stroke is either not changed or is slightly reduced.

The other major benefits of estrogen relate to "quality of life" issues. Hot flashes, night sweats, and vaginal dryness disappear with estrogen replacement. The increase in facial hair often seen with menopause is decreased with estrogen replacement. Genital prolapse is also less likely to occur. Other symptoms that may be alleviated with hormone replacement include insomnia, palpitations, mood disturbances, decreased sex drive, and urinary frequency.

How can I tell if I have osteoporosis, and what can I do to prevent it?

The diagnosis of osteoporosis can be made through a variety of tests that measure bone density. Women who are at risk for getting osteoporosis should consider having a bone density test. These are some of the risk factors that can predispose you to osteoporosis:

- *Small bones:* This condition is usually found in thinner women.

- *Consumption of cigarettes, alcohol, and caffeine:* This is another reason to quit those bad habits. Smoking is particularly hard on bones.

- *Family history of osteoporosis:* Did your mom start to lose height and develop a curvature in her upper back? If so, she had osteoporosis, and you may too.

- *White or Asian race:* Osteoporosis is found less frequently among black women.

- *Inadequate calcium intake:* Women rarely consume adequate amounts of calcium. Peak bone mass is reached by age 35. If your diet was deficient in dairy products before age 35, your risk of osteoporosis is increased substantially.

- *Insufficient exercise:* Bone density is maintained through regular exercise, particularly weight-bearing exercise such as walking, cycling, and dancing.

- *Late onset of menses or early menopause:* Since estrogen protects against bone thinning, girls who begin menstruating late or women who enter menopause early are more at risk for developing osteoporosis.

- *Anorexia:* Women with a history of anorexia are more likely to have low bone density due to inadequate diet and decreased estrogen production.

- *Pregnancy and breast-feeding:* These place extra demands on the calcium in your system. Extra calcium intake is required to meet these demands if bone loss is to be prevented.

- *Certain medications:* These include corticosteroids (anti-inflammatory steroids used in treating asthma and arthritis), anticonvulsants (antiseizure medicines), furosemide diuretics (the "water pill," which is used to treat fluid retention and high blood pressure), and thyroid replacement (for an underactive thyroid gland). If you must take these medications, you should consider taking special measures to decrease bone loss.

Of the currently available methods for assessing bone density, DEXA (dual energy x-ray absorptiometry) scanning is best. If you wish to have your bone density measured, try to find a facility that employs this technique.

A proper diet is important in the prevention of osteoporosis. Teenagers should increase their calcium intake through diet and supplements to 1,500 milligrams per day. The teens are critical bone-building years. Unfortunately, most teenage girls do not drink much milk. The easiest way to combat this problem, if you have a teenage daughter, is to keep a roll of Tums or Rolaids on the dinner table and give her one at each meal.

Women of ages 25 to 50 should take 1,000 milligrams of calcium per day. In menopause the requirements increase again to 1,500 milligrams. Consuming foods rich in calcium is vital. It is, however, almost impossible to consume enough calcium through diet alone. Most women in menopause need to take a calcium supplement to reach the goal. Calcium supplements are available over the counter. Most contain calcium carbonate, as do the antacids Tums and Rolaids. Refer to the product's label to find the amount of elemental calcium (it may be abbreviated Ca++) provided per tablet. Calculate how much calcium you are getting in your diet, and add enough of the supplement to reach the daily goal. Because you can absorb only 750 milligrams of calcium at one time, it is best to divide your supplements and take them throughout the day. Calcium carbonate is best absorbed when taken with a little food or orange juice. Vitamin D is also critical to calcium absorption and bone mineralization. Most people get sufficient vitamin D from exposure to the sun or through diet (fatty fish, butter, egg yolks, liver, and fortified milk supply this vitamin). If you don't drink milk or get out in the sun much, consider taking a supplement. Some calcium supple-

Foods Containing Calcium

	Amount	Calcium (milligrams)	Fat (grams)
Cheese	1 ounce	150–220	6–9
Cottage cheese	1 cup	210	9.5
Hard ice cream	1 cup	175	14
Milk	1 cup	300	whole, 8; low-fat, 5; skim, 1
Low-fat yogurt	1 cup	350–400	2.5–3.5
Almonds	1 ounce	66	16
Scallops, steamed	3 1/2 ounce	115	1.4
Shrimp, raw	3 1/2 ounce	63	0.8
Broccoli, cooked	2/3 cup	88	0.3
Spinach, cooked	1/2 cup	83	0.3
Kale, cooked	3/4 cup	187	0.7
Turnip greens, cooked	2/3 cup	184	0.2
Beans, canned	1/2 cup	68	3.2
Green beans, cooked	1 cup	62	0.2
Chickpeas (garbanzos)	3 1/2 oz	75	2.4
Sweet potato, baked	1 small	40	0.5
Figs, dried	5 medium	126	1.3
Raisins	5/8 cup	62	0.2
Orange	1 medium	56	0.1

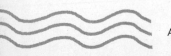

ments also contain vitamin D, as do multivitamins. The recommended daily allowance is 400 IU. The nearby table can help you calculate how much calcium you obtain from the foods you eat.

Exercise effectively slows bone loss during menopause. Some studies indicate that it may even be able to increase bone density. The best exercises are weight-bearing in nature, such as walking, bicycling, dancing, step climbing, and weight lifting. Exercise also helps develop muscles and maintains a healthy heart.

Although estrogen is the most effective means of slowing or stopping bone loss in menopause, other agents can be used to treat osteoporosis. Bisphosphonates are a group of drugs that inhibit bone breakdown. A new bisphosphonate called alendronate (Fosamax) is effective at preventing fractures. Fosamax is probably the most widely used nonhormonal medication for the prevention and treatment of osteoporosis, but it is a bit of a pain in the neck. You must take it with a full glass of water when you get up in the morning, then you must stay upright and cannot eat or drink anything for at least 30 to 45 minutes. Some people develop gastrointestinal distress from Fosamax. If you have a history of heartburn or gastritis, Fosamax may not be your best bet.

Given by injection or nasal spray, calcitonin (Calcimar, Cibacalcin, and Miacalcin) decreases the breakdown of bone. It also appears to relieve pain for women with bone fractures. Calcitonin may not be as effective as estrogen or alendronate in preventing bone loss, but it appears to be safe and is usually well tolerated.

Sodium fluoride has also been shown to increase bone density, though studies have demonstrated that the new bone produced by sodium fluoride is structurally weaker than normal bone. Used in conjunction with calcium, a slow-release form of sodium fluoride appears to reduce fracture rates.

All of these medications have risks associated with their use. Your doctor can help you decide if any are appropriate for you. You can also obtain information from this organization:

National Osteoporosis Foundation
1150 17th Street NW

Suite 500
Washington, DC 20036
(202) 223-2226
www.nof.org

What type of hormone should I take? How are they given?

Almost all the benefits of hormonal replacement derive from estrogen. However, estrogen taken without progesterone increases the risk of developing endometrial cancer, so women who have not undergone hysterectomy must also take progesterone to counteract the effects of estrogen on the endometrium. Women who have decreased sex drive, fatigue, or a diminished sense of well-being may benefit from the addition of testosterone. Testosterone also helps reduce breast tenderness, a common problem with hormone replacement.

Estrogen replacement usually takes the form of tablets, capsules, or skin patches. The tablets are usually taken daily. The patch is changed once or twice weekly. Patients who get gastrointestinal distress from the tablets may do better with the patch; the same goes for women with gallbladder disease, headaches, high blood pressure, high triglycerides, or diabetes. Women who get skin reactions from the patch may prefer tablets. Women who use estrogen primarily to relieve vaginal symptoms may benefit most from vaginal creams or the vaginal estrogen ring. The estrogen ring (Estring), a flexible ring placed into the vagina, delivers a low dose of estrogen to the vagina and bladder without substantially affecting other areas of the body. It remains in place (without interfering with intercourse) and is changed by the patient or doctor every three months.

Traditionally, the most common estrogen used in replacement regimens has been Premarin, which is actually a composite of many estrogens derived from the urine of pregnant horses. Most studies that have evaluated the effects of estrogen on women involved the use of Premarin. Other physicians prefer to use estrogens similar to those found naturally in women. These are either synthesized or obtained from plant sources. Each doctor tends to have a preference, and no good evidence proves that one brand is superior to all others. Most hormonal regimens provide estrogen continuously. Some doctors have the patient

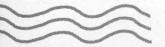

stop taking the estrogen for five to seven days each month although no evidence suggests that this is necessary.

There is more variation in how physicians prescribe progesterone. Women who have had a hysterectomy usually do not need this hormone. In certain situations, such as hormone replacement after hysterectomy for endometriosis (see page 112), progesterone may also be given. There are two basic regimens for giving progesterone. The cyclic one provides progesterone for 10 to 14 days each month. The woman typically gets a menstrual period after the progesterone is stopped each month, but will not become pregnant. This regimen emulates a normal menstrual cycle. It has been the standard in hormone replacement for the past two decades.

Because many women aren't thrilled with the prospect of resuming menstruation, many physicians have switched to a continuous regimen, in which a smaller amount of progesterone is taken every day. Up to 40 percent of women will experience erratic bleeding initially on this regimen. But by the end of the first year, 80 percent of women will no longer have any bleeding. Both progesterone regimens are equally beneficial. If you can tolerate unpredictable bleeding for a few months (or more), try the continuous regimen. If you think erratic bleeding will be distressing, you're better off with a cyclic regimen. Some physicians use a combination of the two regimens.

The most common progesterone prescribed is medroxyprogesterone (Provera, Cycrin). However, others may be used to provide similar protection to the endometrium. Natural progesterone may also be given, particularly to those women who experience side effects from the synthetic progestins. Because natural progesterone is more expensive, shows greater variability, and is absorbed more erratically, most doctors prefer the synthetic type.

Do I have to wait until I stop getting periods to begin hormone replacement therapy?

You are still getting fairly regular periods but have noticed progressively worsening hot flashes and night sweats. Perhaps your mood swings are "off the chart." You're wondering if this could be menopause, but your doctor says, "No it isn't, because you are still getting periods." To be fair, you both are correct. By definition, you are still producing pre-menopausal levels of estrogen. You will no longer menstruate when your estrogen level falls into the menopausal range. If your body is making less estrogen than previously, however, you can still experience menopausal symptoms. If the symptoms are severe, there is no reason to put off hormonal supplementation as long as the doses of estrogen and progesterone are balanced. Some physicians will provide hormonal supplementation in a fashion similar to the cyclic regimen discussed under the previous question. Others will recommend taking low-dose oral contraceptives unless there is a medical reason for avoiding them (see page 39). Oral contraceptives are a particularly good choice if you also have either heavy or irregular periods.

Is there an age at which it is too late to start hormone replacement therapy?

The ideal time to start is immediately following menopause. The most rapid bone loss occurs in the ten years after onset. For the most part, lost bone can't be regained and plaque in the coronary arteries doesn't go away. Nevertheless, estrogen replacement does appear to have protective effects for bones and heart even when treatment is started later in life. If you are at risk for osteoporosis or heart disease, consider beginning hormone replacement therapy even if you are making a late start.

I don't want to take hormones because they cause cancer. Am I right?

It is especially important to separate myth from reality when analyzing the risk of cancer related to hormone replacement therapy. One of the most common reasons that women give for refusing hormone replacement therapy is the concern about getting cancer. Two different potential risks exist: uterine cancer and breast cancer. Let's look at each of them separately.

The risk of getting uterine cancer is very clearly understood. If you take estrogen by itself, your risk of developing endometrial cancer (cancer of the inside lining of the uterus) is increased up to fourfold. It is equally clear that if you take enough progesterone with your estrogen, this increased risk can be *eliminated*. We want to make this absolutely clear. It is often said that the risk can be *decreased* with the addition of progesterone, leading one to assume that there is still an increased risk. This is misleading. With proper dosing, progesterone reduces risk to the point at which it is no greater (and it even may be less) than the risk of getting endometrial cancer without hormone replacement. The most commonly used progesterone is medroxyprogesterone (Provera, Cycrin). Taking five to ten milligrams of medroxyprogesterone for 12 to 14 days each month offers adequate protection. A dose of two and a half milligrams daily is also sufficient in a continuous regimen. If you or your doctor chooses not to include progesterone in your hormone replacement, annual surveillance of the endometrium with endometrial biopsies and/or ultrasound scans is mandatory. Women who have undergone hysterectomy do not require progesterone as part of hormone replacement, since there is no longer a risk of developing endometrial cancer.

Does estrogen replacement increase the risk of getting breast cancer?

It's hard to believe, but the answer is still not clear. Many studies that have addressed this issue have not found an increased relative risk of breast cancer related to estrogen replacement. However, other studies have concluded that an increased risk of breast cancer occurs with long-term use (more than five years). Most studies have concluded that there is no increased risk with short-term use (less than five years).

Why is there no definitive answer after many years of research? Most studies were done at a time when dosages and hormonal regimens differed from those in use today. Because different studies focus on different populations, comparing their results does not provide conclusive, widely applicable information.

So what can a poor soul conclude from this? It is easy to be confused by terms like *relative risk*. You really want the answer to this question: "What are *my* chances of getting breast cancer if I take these hormones?" For every 100 women using estrogen for more than 10 years, 3 more may develop cancer than would normally do so. If you are at high risk for developing breast cancer (see page 160), estrogen replacement may not be in your best interest. You must weigh this risk against that of developing coronary heart disease or osteoporosis. Most women are at far greater risk of dying from a heart attack than from breast cancer, and for most, the benefits of hormone replacement outweigh the risks. A definitive answer may come in the year 2005, when the Women's Health Initiative is expected to release the results of a clinical trial. Until then, consult with your doctor.

What side effects will I get from hormone replacement?

The two most common complaints we hear from women beginning hormone replacement therapy are bleeding and breast tenderness. We have already talked about what might be expected in terms of bleeding (see page 175). Breast tenderness is another common complaint. It is most likely to be a problem for those who have had severe premenstrual breast tenderness before menopause. The tenderness usually disappears after menopause, only to return when hormone replacement is started. Breast enlargement may also occur. Breast tenderness from hormone replacement sometimes tapers off over time. Decreasing caffeine intake and taking supplemental vitamin E (400 to 800 IU per day) may help (see page 154). If the tenderness is severe, adding a small amount of testosterone to the hormone regimen or reducing the dose of estrogen may help.

You may experience gastrointestinal distress, including nausea, cramping, and bloating, as a side effect of hormone replacement. These symptoms tend to wane over time. The symptoms may also be reduced by changing to a different brand of estrogen or to a different way of taking it, such as through a patch instead of in tablets.

Less common side effects include headaches, mood disturbance, skin changes (particularly a spotty darkening of the skin when it is exposed to the sun), and fluid retention. Developing gallbladder disease is also more likely on hormone replacement therapy.

You're probably ready to give up on trying hormone replacement after hearing about these side effects. *Remember that most women tolerate hormone replacement with few or no side effects.* You are far more likely to experience beneficial effects — decreased hot flashes and night sweats, no vaginal dryness, less frequent urination, improved sleep, better mood — rather than detrimental effects. If you do develop a side effect that cannot be managed, you can always discontinue the therapy.

Aren't those hormones going to make me gain weight?

You may gain weight, but it won't be caused by the hormone replacement. Many women will get heavier at this time of life, whether or not they use hormone replacement. As your activity level decreases and your metabolic rate slows, weight may increase. You must either eat less and reduce your consumption of fatty foods or exercise more to keep your weight stable.

Are there women who can't take hormones?

Some women are not good candidates for hormone replacement therapy. Traditionally, women with a history of breast or endometrial cancer cannot use hormone replacement, since the risk of recurrence may be increased if estrogen is given. Recently, physicians have begun to consider hormone replacement for women whose cancer was caught at a very early stage, suggesting that the risk of recurrence is low. Women who have been free of disease for a long time, usually at least five to ten years, may also be potential candidates. Still, prescribing hormones for women who have had either of these cancers is very controversial, and most physicians will not do so.

In addition, most physicians will not prescribe hormone replacement for women who have had deep-vein thrombosis (DVT), or blood clots in the large veins of the legs. (This rule does not apply to superficial veins that are readily visible.) Clots in the deep veins can travel to the lungs, a potentially life-threatening situation, and estrogen may affect blood clotting.

Active liver disease (hepatitis) may also rule out the use of hormones, since estrogen is metabolized (eliminated from the system) by the liver.

If you currently have gallbladder disease or if you have gallstones, hormone replacement may not be in your best interest. This disadvantage must be weighed against the benefits that the hormones will provide to your heart and bones. You can, however, get along fine without your gallbladder. You can't do well with a damaged heart or crumbling bones.

In the past, doctors didn't recommend hormone replacement for women with diabetes (high blood sugar) and hypertension (high blood pressure). Research has shown, however, that estrogen replacement does not worsen these conditions. Because both conditions can put a woman at risk for coronary heart disease, hormone replacement should be considered because it offers protection against heart disease.

Other than hormones, what can I take to alleviate my symptoms?

What can you do if you or your physician decides that hormone replacement is not an option, but you have problematic menopausal symptoms? Bellargal and clonidine are two nonhormonal medications that can treat hot flashes when taking estrogen isn't wise.

Taken in tablet form twice a day, Bellargal combines a sedative with medications that decrease the activity of the part of the nervous system that modulates sweating and flushing. It is not recommended for women with coronary heart disease (a history of heart attack or angina), diseases of the blood vessels, high blood pressure, glaucoma, or kidney or liver dysfunction. It also must be used carefully for those who take antiseizure, anticoagulant, or antidepressant medications. Bellargal is usually tolerated well, but occasional side effects include tingling, blurry vision, palpitations, dry mouth, decreased sweating, constipation, urinary retention (inability to empty the bladder), and drowsiness.

Traditionally used for high blood pressure, clonidine (Catapres) has also been prescribed more recently as a treatment for hot flashes and night sweats. It is administered either orally or as a patch (changed weekly). Side effects are usually mild and diminish with continued use. They include nausea, fatigue, headache, dizziness, and nervousness. Clonidine must be used cautiously in patients with severe coronary (heart) or cerebral (brain) vascular disease.

We're often asked about the use of "natural" products for the treatment of hot flashes. Numerous plants have estrogen-like substances

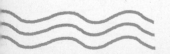

called phytoestrogens, and advocates of "natural medicine" claim that they are safer to use than prescription estrogens. Foods high in phytoestrogens include soybeans and soybean products, such as soy milk and tofu. Phytoestrogens are also derived from some vegetables and berries as well as grains, seeds, and sprouts. Preliminary evidence suggests that foods high in phytoestrogens can help relieve menopausal symptoms while lowering the risk of breast cancer. Phytoestrogens are worthy of further evaluation, and their potential is exciting. But they have not yet been evaluated carefully enough to warrant fully embracing them as alternatives to hormone replacement therapy.

"Natural" progesterone products have received much publicity. Many creams are available over the counter today. Some contain micronized progesterone (a natural progesterone derived from plants), and others are made with wild yam extracts, which manufacturers claim have progesterone-like effects. Using such progesterone creams as a substitute for prescribed progesterone in a hormone replacement regimen can be dangerous; there is no evidence that these products can adequately balance the effects of estrogen in the endometrium. There is no pathway by which the human body can convert wild yam extracts to progesterone. Micronized progesterone can be absorbed, but you'd need a lot of cream to achieve progesterone levels comparable to those found during a normal menstrual cycle. Progesterone creams will not provide the medical benefits attributed to estrogen replacement therapy.

Vitamins are often recommended for the treatment of hot flashes and night sweats. Vitamin E, in doses ranging from 400 to 1,600 milligrams per day, has been reported to help relieve hot flashes. There is a dearth of scientific studies to substantiate this claim, but you can try it. As an antioxidant, vitamin E is thought to be valuable. It may help the body clear itself of harmful byproducts (called free radicals) that cause cellular damage. Many scientists feel that antioxidants decrease the risk of developing vascular disease and cancer, although this benefit has not been conclusively proved.

Changes in lifestyle may help in coping with hot flashes. Some women say their menopausal symptoms are worse when they are under stress. Other women experience more hot flashes when they eat hot or spicy food and drinks. Regular exercise may also reduce menopausal symptoms and generally enhance well-being.

What are those new drugs that are supposed to replace estrogen, and are they safer?

Imagine a drug that has all the benefits of estrogen but none of the risks. It protects your bones, reduces your risk of heart disease, and douses those hot flashes without any potentially negative effects on your breasts or uterus. Although no such drug exists, scientists are currently developing compounds called SERMs (selective estrogen receptor modulators) that aspire to meet those lofty goals. SERMs mimic the effects of estrogen in some areas of the body, while blocking them in others.

Raloxifene (Evista) is the first SERM to gain FDA approval. It appears to prevent osteoporosis and to reduce the risk of getting coronary heart disease without causing adverse effects on the breasts or uterus. It sounds great, so what's the catch? It isn't as effective as estrogen in preventing bone thinning and heart disease. It also may increase the frequency — although not the severity — of hot flashes, which estrogen eliminates. Although raloxifene is not a panacea, it does appear to provide another choice for women. Certainly more SERMs will follow, which is encouraging news for women everywhere.

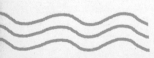

14 Where's the Nearest Bathroom?

Why do I always have to run to the bathroom?

Scene: Turnpike

Gladys: "When's the next rest stop?"

Harry: "Why?"

Gladys: "I have to go to the bathroom."

Harry: "Didn't you just go?"

Gladys: "Yeah, but I have to go again."

Harry: "Can't you wait until you get home?"

Does this exchange sound familiar? It seems as if you're always running to the bathroom. You know where they're all located, even the disgusting one behind the butcher counter in the supermarket. Your children have started to kid you about it.

You may have an unstable bladder. This condition is also referred to as an irritable, or spastic, bladder. An unstable bladder makes you go to the bathroom more often and gives you that sense of urgency. When severe, it is associated with incontinence; you start to lose urine before you can make it to the bathroom. The unwanted bladder contractions may occur spontaneously or be triggered by the sound of running water. The uninhibited contractions may be caused by an infection, stones in the bladder, or a deficiency of estrogen. They can also result from diseases that affect the nervous system, such as stroke or Parkinson's disease. Most often, though, there is no identifiable source.

If you have incontinence, you should see a gynecologist, urologist, or gynecologic urologist. Some conditions can be diagnosed only with testing.

URINARY PROBLEMS

If no obvious cause is found, try eliminating caffeine (contained in coffee, tea, chocolate, colas) and alcohol from your diet. They act like diuretics ("water pills"), causing the bladder to fill more rapidly than usual and inducing spasms. If you take a prescribed diuretic, ask your doctor if you can replace it with a different type of medication or reduce the amount. If you must take a diuretic, time the doses for when you will be at home.

Now that you've rid yourself of the culprits that worsen your condition, you can work on controlling your bladder instead of letting it control you. To start, choose a time interval that you can successfully wait between voidings — anywhere from half an hour on up. If you choose to wait for an hour, throughout one week go to the bathroom every hour on the hour and empty your bladder. If you are successful — without any accidents — add 15 minutes to the waiting time for the next week. Every week that you are successful, add 15 more minutes until you get to a reasonable interval, at least three to four hours. This method of training really does work, *but* (and this is a big *but*) you have to be motivated to follow through with it. You do *not* have to wake yourself up during the night to comply with the schedule, however.

Another goal is to learn how to control the sense of urgency until it subsides. Don't submit to your first impulse to run to the bathroom. Stop what you are doing and remain still. Squeeze your pelvic muscles (see page 186) several times, to prevent leakage. Sit down, if possible, and try to relax and release tension. Taking a few slow, deep breaths may help. Remain calm and focus on letting the urge subside. When it does, you can resume other activities or walk to the bathroom slowly, continuing to squeeze your pelvic muscles. The idea is to regain control over your bladder, not vice versa.

If you are menopausal, estrogen replacement therapy may reduce your sense of urinary urgency and frequency. Estrogen sustains the inside lining of the bladder and urethra. Without estrogen, the lining atrophies, producing increased urination, a feeling of urgency, and burning. Estrogen replacement therapy will reverse these changes. Even small amounts of estrogen cream applied to the vagina can help.

When all else fails, your doctor can prescribe a medication that can help reduce bladder irritability. Unfortunately, there's a catch (isn't there always!). Most of them have annoying side effects, the most common of which is dry mouth. Sucking hard candy or chewing gum may help. Other side effects include palpitations, constipation, blurry vision, and decreased perspiration. Women with glaucoma, unstable heart disease, or conditions associated with blockage of the bowel or bladder should avoid these medications.

Is it normal to get up at night to go to the bathroom?

Getting up once is not unusual. More often than that is not typical, however. There are several reasons for this problem. First, many people consume beverages in the late evening because it may be the first time all day to sit down and relax. Others do so because they don't drink enough liquid in the daytime, and they make up the difference in the evening. Try to drink more throughout the day and restrict the amounts of fluids consumed at night, particularly caffeinated and alcoholic beverages, which have diuretic properties. Do not take a prescribed diuretic ("water pill") within two to three hours of bedtime. Women with an unstable bladder (see page 183) will also experience nighttime frequency and urgency.

Fluid that has been retained throughout the day may also cause frequent urination at night. It appears as swelling in the legs, particularly the ankles and feet. When you lie down at night, the fluid makes its way out of the legs and up to the kidneys, where it is eliminated, causing those extra trips to the bathroom. A prescribed diuretic taken at dinnertime may help the kidneys excrete the retained fluid before bedtime. Consult your doctor to rule out more serious conditions that cause fluid retention.

Why do I lose urine when I cough or sneeze?

Losing urine with a cough, sneeze, or laugh is common and is referred to as urinary stress incontinence (USI). It is usually caused by inadequate support where the urethra enters the bladder. Childbirth, age, menopause, and a lifetime of lifting and pushing have conspired to destroy the support in this region. Even your genes may have betrayed you. Fair-skinned women of northern European origin and Asian women have a particularly high likelihood of developing stress incontinence.

Other stresses that may produce incontinence include running, jumping, and dancing.

Luckily, you can improve your continence by strengthening the muscles of the pelvic floor. First you need to identify which muscles to work on. Place one or two fingers in your vagina. Now squeeze the pelvic muscles until you feel them tighten around your finger. This is the same muscle group that enables you to voluntarily shut off your stream of urine (this may help you identify the correct muscles). Try to contract them without tightening your abdominal muscles. Place your other hand on your abdomen to make sure that it remains soft while you contract the muscles. Squeeze the muscles for a count of three, then relax them for a count of three. Repeat this exercise 15 times during one session. Try to do three sessions daily. When you can reliably identify the correct muscles, you can do these exercises, which are called Kegel exercises, without your fingers inside. You can do them while waiting in line for the train or while sitting at a traffic light. As long as you're not grimacing, who's to know?

Several devices, used in conjunction with physical therapy provided by a gynecologic physical therapist, a gynecologist, or a nurse, can maximize the benefits of these exercises. For example, a manometer, which registers the amount of pressure generated by squeezing the pelvic support muscles, can provide feedback. Tamponlike devices, called weighted vaginal cones, are also useful. You place a cone in the vagina and keep it there for 15 minutes, twice daily, by tightening your pelvic support muscles. The weight of the cone is increased until you can successfully retain the heaviest one. In another treatment, an electrical cylinder is placed in the vagina, where it delivers an electrical impulse that contracts the pelvic support muscles.

Exercises often help this condition, particularly mild stress incontinence. But unfortunately, much of the support for the bladder and urethra is obtained from fibrous tissue. Fibrous tissue that is torn or stretched cannot be restored without surgery. A healthy diet and estrogen replacement after menopause may help maintain the integrity of this tissue, but most of its strength is predetermined by genetics: You're either born with strong tissue or you're not.

Mechanical devices may be used to improve bladder control. They are especially useful when incontinence is associated with a specific activity such as running, aerobic exercise, or dancing. They are put in place before the activity is begun and removed afterward. They include Introl, a rubber device shaped much like a diaphragm but set with a forked prong that fits under the urethra. It has the drawback of being expensive ($300). Some women have success using a tampon or a pessary (see page 193); some pessaries are designed specifically to manage stress incontinence and cost only $30 to $40. Reliance, a balloon-tipped insert that inflates to block the urethra, may also help. Impress, a tiny foam pad placed over the opening of the urethra and held in place by an adhesive gel, also controls incontinence.

If conservative measures don't work, surgery is recommended. Urologic evaluation prior to surgery is strongly recommended. If you have genuine stress incontinence, your chances that surgery will solve the problem are great. If your incontinence is related to other causes, such as an unstable bladder, the surgery will not be successful. In fact, surgery may make the problem worse.

Stress incontinence may also be related to an intrinsic defect in the urethral sphincter mechanism. The urethral sphincter comprises the muscles in the wall of the urethra where it passes into the bladder. If these muscles don't keep the urethra closed, urine will be lost when an activity increases pressure in the abdomen (laughing, coughing, sneezing). This defect cannot be corrected by the standard surgical techniques used for stress incontinence. Medications containing either phenylpropanolamine (such as Ornade) or pseudoephedrine (Sudafed) can strengthen urethral tone. You can try an over-the-counter decongestant or appetite suppressant that contains these medications, but they must be used cautiously if you have high blood pressure, cardiac disease, or hyperthyroidism. Side effects include palpitations, nervousness, headaches, and insomnia.

Doctors can also inject collagen (the stuff that makes up fibrous tissue) directly into the wall of the urethra to correct its structural defects. These injections help the urethra close more effectively. Often, repeated injections are necessary to obtain optimal benefit. If collagen injections are not successful, the doctor may recommend a "sling" surgical procedure, in which a sling of tissue (either natural or synthetic) is placed under the urethra at the bladder to support and close the urethra.

For more information on incontinence, consider the following resources:

National Association for Continence
P.O. Box 8310
Spartanburg, SC 29305
800-BLADDER

Continence Restored, Inc.
407 Strawberry Hill Avenue
Stamford, CT 06902
(914) 285-1470 or
(204) 348-0601

Why do I keep getting bladder infections?

Bladder infection, or cystitis, is fairly common. The opening of the bladder (the urethral meatus) is located just above the opening of the vagina. Since the vagina contains many bacteria, it is not surprising that these organisms gain access to the bladder. Intercourse often provides such an opportunity. Increased sexual activity often gives rise to "honeymoon cystitis."

An occasional bout of cystitis can be treated by taking antibiotics and forcing fluids. Ideally, you should have a urine culture performed if you have symptoms of infection, since not all infections respond to the same antibiotic. Recurrent bladder infections should prompt your doctor to order additional studies. Get urine cultures every time there is an infection. A repeat culture should be obtained two weeks after finishing the antibiotics. If the same bacteria are still present after treatment, then they probably did not respond to the original antibiotic. If the infection appears to clear each time, the problem is reinfection.

Frequent reinfection (three to four times per year) may be a sign of a more serious underlying condition. You should see a urologist for additional studies. You may have a congenital defect in your urinary tract, bladder (or kidney) stones, or a diverticulum (a sac or pouch opening out from the bladder wall). The doctor will probably perform tests to evaluate your urethra and your bladder function. Often no source for the recurrent infections is found. In that situation, you may be given a low dose of an antibiotic daily or sometimes less frequently to prevent future infections.

What can I do to avoid recurrent infections?

If your infections are being induced by sexual activity, it may help to empty your bladder after intercourse. If you are not sufficiently lubricated during intercourse, your urethra can be injured, so you may want to use a sterile lubricant, such as K-Y jelly. If you get recurrent infections, make sure you drink plenty of liquids throughout the day and empty your bladder on a regular basis. A compound in cranberry juice inhibits bacterial growth. After voiding, wipe only from front to back. Good hygiene is essential in preventing recurrent infections. You and your partner need to keep the genital and anal areas clean. Showers are better than baths. Avoid tight clothing, and wear cotton rather than synthetic fabrics. Synthetics trap heat and moisture (a lovely environment for bacteria), whereas cotton breathes. In postmenopausal women, estrogen replacement may help prevent recurrent infections (see chapter 13 for more on estrogen replacement).

My doctor says I have interstitial cystitis. What's that?

If you have to urinate frequently with great urgency and have pain in your pelvis or just above your pubic bone and no obvious cause has been identified, you may have interstitial cystitis, an inflammatory bladder disorder that is not caused by infection with bacteria. Nobody knows for sure what causes it, and women often have symptoms for years before an accurate diagnosis is made.

The diagnosis of interstitial cystitis is usually made by cystoscopy. While you're under anesthesia, a telescopic instrument is introduced into the bladder through the urethra. A bladder biopsy may be taken and sent for analysis. These tests may reveal the bladder to be ulcerated or inflamed.

No single treatment for interstitial cystitis has been found to work for everybody. Some foods and beverages appear to aggravate the

URINARY PROBLEMS

symptoms. Alcohol, beverages containing caffeine, chocolate, citrus fruits, tomatoes, and spicy foods seem to be the prime offenders. Bladder training (see page 184) will also help some women. Other conservative measures include stress management and biofeedback. A new drug, Elmiron, recently approved by the FDA, has been found to relieve symptoms in nearly 40 percent of patients. Antidepressants and antihistamines give varying degrees of success. Approximately 90 percent of women will eventually respond to treatment with medication.

When drug treatment fails, surgery may be recommended. Enlarging the bladder may help reduce urinary frequency and urgency. When symptoms are severe and intractable, urinary division can be performed. In this procedure, urine is diverted to a pouch constructed from intestinal tissue.

Interstitial cystitis is a frustrating condition. You may have symptoms for years before an accurate diagnosis is rendered and may try various treatment regimens without significant or lasting improvement. Be persistent in exploring a variety of treatments, and remember that most women will ultimately find relief.

For further information on interstitial cystitis, we suggest you consult this organization:

The Interstitial Cystitis Association
P.O. Box 1553
Madison Square Station
New York, NY 10159
(212) 979-6057
http://www.ichelp.com

15 Pelvic Prolapse: The "Dropped Bladder"

What is that bulge down there?

You were feeling perfectly fine. Then one day you feel a mass bulging when you wipe yourself, and you're scared out of your wits! Your first thought is that you must have a tumor. It's much more likely that you have pelvic prolapse, also called pelvic descensus or pelvic relaxation, the descent of the pelvic organs due to inadequate support. The most common of these problems is cystocele, or "dropped bladder," the descent of the bladder down the vagina. Other problems can include a rectocele (the descent of the rectum into the vagina), uterine descensus (dropped uterus), vaginal vault prolapse (in which the vagina turns inside out and protrudes), and enterocele (herniation between the walls of the vagina and rectum).

The uterus, bladder, and rectum are supported by fibrous tissue (also called connective tissue) and ligaments (not as firm as the ligaments that are in joints). They are also supported by muscles that make up the floor of the pelvis, referred to as the pelvic diaphragm. Stretching and tearing of tissues during childbirth can result in permanent damage to these structures. A lifetime of straining and pushing and lifting heavy objects also places stress on them. Connective tissue deteriorates with age and menopause. Over time, cumulative stress can produce pelvic prolapse.

White women, especially northern Europeans, Egyptians, and women from India, are particularly susceptible to this condition, which appears less frequently in other Asian and black women. If your mother has pelvic support problems, your risk of experiencing it is increased.

What symptoms will I have from prolapse?

Symptoms vary according to the size and type of defect. Mild to moderate relaxation of pelvic support is common and usually not associated with any symptoms. As the prolapse progresses, a bulging sensation or pressure in the lower vagina can be felt. Some women liken this sensation to "sitting on an egg." A "pulling" or cramping in the lower abdomen, groin, pelvis, and lower back may also be experienced. These symptoms are usually accentuated by standing and lifting. Difficulty in emptying the bladder may accompany this condition, and it may give rise to frequent bladder infections.

I lose my urine. Is that because of my dropped bladder?

Patients and doctors often incorrectly attribute incontinence to a dropped bladder, but by itself it does not usually cause incontinence. If you have incontinence, don't assume that it is related to this condition. The incontinence must be evaluated as a separate condition (see chapter 14).

Is pelvic prolapse dangerous? What can I do to keep it from getting worse?

Minor degrees of pelvic prolapse do not require aggressive intervention; there is no particular danger. The muscles that provide support to the rectum, vagina, and bladder can be strengthened through the exercises described on page 184.

If you are postmenopausal, you should consider hormone replacement therapy if you have pelvic prolapse, since estrogen prevents atrophy of the lining of the vagina and strengthens the pelvic connective tissue.

If you have pelvic prolapse, refrain from heavy lifting, pushing, and pulling. Any activity that increases abdominal pressure is likely to worsen your condition. When lifting an object, use your legs rather than your abdominal muscles to bear weight. Squat close to the object, and straighten your legs as you lift it. Fill your grocery bags and laundry baskets half full. Avoid carrying the grandchildren. Place them on the couch next to you if you want to snuggle. If you go for a walk, place

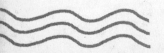

the child in a stroller. Stop moving furniture when you clean. Get your children or husband to do it. While you're at it, have them lug that heavy vacuum cleaner upstairs.

Medical conditions that induce chronic coughing or constipation may worsen pelvic prolapse. You and your doctor should try to correct them, if possible. Losing weight may also be of benefit if you are very heavy. If you have not already done so, stop smoking. Do not wear a girdle. The girdle increases pressure on the abdomen, placing downward pressure on the pelvic organs.

How is prolapse corrected?

When prolapse has progressed beyond the opening of the vagina, it is unlikely that exercises or other therapeutic techniques will be of much benefit. You must proceed with surgical correction or using a pessary. A rubber device inserted into the vagina, the pessary provides support to the pelvic organs. Ring-shaped pessaries are most common, but other shapes are also available. Some pessaries are inserted and removed by the doctor. Others are designed to permit self-insertion and removal.

The pessary is fitted in the doctor's office. It should not be uncomfortable and should relieve some of the pressure you were experiencing from the prolapse. Because the pessary is a foreign object, it may cause a discharge, often foul smelling, to develop. Trimo-san, an acidic vaginal gel, may be used with a pessary to decrease the discharge. Returning to the doctor's office on a regular basis — approximately every three months — will be required. At that time the doctor will remove the pessary, clean it, and also clean the vagina and inspect it for any sign of ulceration. Postmenopausal women can decrease the likelihood of developing vaginal ulceration by taking estrogen replacement therapy. Even small amounts of estrogen cream can help. Pessaries that are self-inserted are less likely to cause abnormal discharge or vaginal ulceration. Usually, it is inserted in the morning and removed at night. It can also be removed for intercourse.

Surgery is the most definitive approach to correcting prolapse. The type of surgery varies according to the type of prolapse. Consult your doctor to assess which might be appropriate for you. It is important that your doctor perform a thorough examination prior to surgery to identify any coexisting bladder problems. Go to the office with a full bladder. The doctor can elevate the bladder with his or her fingers, simulating a surgical repair, and can check for stress incontinence while you cough. Many gynecologists recommend urologic evaluation before surgery. This examination should be mandatory if you have any symptoms of bladder dysfunction (urgency or frequency of urination, incontinence).

So how do you choose between a pessary and surgery? If your general health is good and you are looking for a permanent solution to the problem, you should probably proceed with surgery. If you want to avoid the risk of undergoing surgery, you're better off trying a pessary. If you don't like it, you can always change your mind and proceed with surgery. Women with severe medical problems should try the pessary.

I hear that surgery doesn't always work. Why?

Most reconstructive surgery for pelvic prolapse succeeds. Most repairs hold up well over time. However, there are no guarantees with this type of surgery. Nobody can predict whether prolapse will recur after surgery.

If your gynecologist is not experienced in vaginal surgery, ask for a referral to someone else. However, certain factors are beyond the control of your doctor. If your connective tissue is particularly weak, the surgery may fail. After surgery, be sure to modify activities that are likely to cause recurrence of the prolapse.

Should I have surgery if I want to have more children?

Ideally, you should postpone surgery until you have completed childbearing. Childbirth will damage the reconstructed pelvic support. Pelvic muscle exercises and pessaries may provide you with enough relief to get by in the meantime.

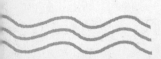

16 When You Need Surgery

What are the complications of surgery?

Do you know the definition of "minor surgery"? It's surgery performed on somebody else. It doesn't matter what anyone says: If you are "going under the knife," it's a big deal. Your concern over potential surgical complications can be healthy. It prompts you to ask your doctor important questions that will better prepare you for surgery. However, don't let your concern evolve into a disabling fear that prevents you from undergoing necessary surgery. Complications that threaten life or necessitate additional surgery are very uncommon in gynecologic surgery. If the benefit of your surgery far outweighs the surgical risks, you should proceed with the operation.

How long will I be in the hospital?

Hospital stays have dramatically decreased in duration over the past few years. Procedures such as D&Cs (dilation and curettage), laparoscopy, and hysteroscopy are usually performed as outpatient surgery. Hospitalization for reconstructive vaginal surgery (see page 194) and major abdominal surgery, such as abdominal hysterectomy, can be as short as two days. It is extended only if there is a severe postoperative complication (as defined by your insurance carrier). You may still need help after you are discharged. Social service and visiting nurse personnel at the hospital can help you make these arrangements. Ask your doctor if home-care services will be necessary. Family members may be able to provide the care. If not, consider contacting the social service department of the hospital before you are admitted. If there will be difficulty in arranging home care,

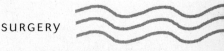

SURGERY

it's easier to solve the problem in advance rather than on the day of discharge.

Will I be "knocked out" during surgery, or can I have a local anesthetic?

The type of surgery dictates which anesthesia is chosen. Some minor procedures can be performed under local anesthesia. Most gynecologic surgery, however, is performed under general anesthesia, which is administered intravenously, or regional anesthesia, which is given in the form of spinal or epidural anesthetics.

General anesthesia will render you completely unconscious. While you are "asleep," an anesthesiologist (or, more commonly, a nurse anesthetist) inserts an endotracheal tube down your windpipe to help you breathe and to protect you from aspirating (accidentally breathing stomach secretions into your lungs). When surgery is finished, the anesthetic agents are discontinued and you will "wake up." Sometimes medications are given to reverse the effects of the anesthesia. If an endotracheal tube was used, it will be withdrawn when you are alert enough to breathe on your own (it may cause you to have a sore throat for a few days). You may feel nauseous from the anesthesia. This problem clears up on its own, but medications can be given if the nausea is severe.

General anesthesia has a low incidence of complications in healthy women. If your surgery involves general anesthesia, you will be instructed to refrain from eating and drinking for at least six hours before surgery, to allow your stomach to empty. General anesthesia may be riskier if you have significant cardiac or pulmonary disease. In these situations, regional or local anesthesia may be preferred.

For regional anesthesia (spinals and epidurals), a needle is inserted near the spinal cord, and "numbing" agents, similar to those used in local anesthesia, are injected to anesthetize the nerves that supply sensation to the lower abdomen and pelvis. Feeling is also lost in the legs. Normal sensation is regained within several hours after surgery. During surgery, the patient remains conscious. Some women like the idea of not having to "go to sleep," whereas others abhor it. If surgery will take a long time, it may become difficult to lie in the same position. Often the anesthesiologist will provide sedation to keep the patient from becoming antsy.

Regional anesthesia does not increase the risk of aspiration. That is its major benefit compared with general anesthesia. It is also safer than general anesthesia for women with significant pulmonary disease (such as asthma). However, some surgeons do not find regional anesthesia satisfactory. If the nerves emanating from the spinal cord are not numbed adequately, some areas may not become completely anesthetized. Anxious patients may find it difficult to remain still and cope with the strange sensations caused by the anesthetic. Individuals with certain spinal or neurologic conditions may not be good candidates for regional anesthesia.

Headaches used to be a concern following regional anesthesia. Patients had to lie flat for 24 hours after surgery and even then might get severe headaches (called spinal headaches) lasting for days or weeks. New techniques, however, have minimized the incidence of spinal headaches, and patients no longer must lie flat after surgery. Injury to the spinal cord from the needle is uncommon. Direct contact of the needle with the spinal cord or the exiting nerves may cause abnormal sensations such as burning, prickling, or numbness in the legs, but these go away spontaneously. Serious adverse reactions to the anesthetics may occur but are rare.

When deemed possible, local anesthesia is usually the safest form of anesthesia, but it can be used only in minor surgery. The choice between regional and general anesthesia is often based on the preference of the anesthesiologist and surgeon. The patient's general health or type of operation may dictate one over the other. Her personal preference may also influence the decision.

If you have concerns regarding your anesthesia, make an appointment with the anesthesiologist before your scheduled date of surgery.

Why do I need a catheter in my bladder?

Immediately before major surgery, after anesthesia has been administered, a rubber catheter is inserted through the urethra into the bladder. A small balloon at one end is inflated with water to prevent the catheter from slipping out. The catheter prevents the bladder from becoming distended with urine during lengthy surgery. It is hooked to a collecting bag that accurately measures urine output; a normal output indicates that blood volume is satisfactory. A low output suggests the need for more intravenous fluids. The catheter is removed the day after surgery. Reconstructive vaginal surgery (see page 194) and bladder suspensions (surgery performed for stress incontinence) require longer catheterization, whereas minor surgical procedures usually do not require catheterization.

What can I get to relieve pain after surgery?

Thanks to modern medicine, you'll experience less pain than women of previous generations. Some operations that used to be performed through large incisions can now be accomplished through small ones with the aid of laparoscopy. Some uterine surgery can be performed through the hysteroscope (see page 92), without any incision. Post-operative pain is diminished with these approaches and can often be controlled with oral painkillers.

There are several approaches to providing relief after major surgery. Traditionally, injections of narcotics were given, usually at four-hour intervals. This is still a reasonable approach for some women. The problem is that pain relief is excellent during the first hour or two after the shot, but diminishes significantly thereafter. By the time your next injection arrives, you may be in considerable pain.

Patient-controlled analgesia (PCA) is a solution to this problem. A narcotic is placed into an intravenous solution and connected to a pump. The patient presses a button to release a small amount of narcotic for pain relief. Pressing the button on a regular basis provides a continuous level of comfort. Overdosing is not possible, because settings on the pump limit the total amount of narcotic that can be released.

Patients undergoing regional anesthesia may have narcotics administered through a catheter left in place near the spinal canal. This treatment is called epidural analgesia. Close monitoring by nursing staff is required for the safe administration of epidural narcotics. When used properly, it provides excellent, sustained pain control after surgery.

Narcotics can produce respiratory and central nervous system depression. Nausea, low blood pressure, and inability to empty the bladder are also potential adverse effects. Intramuscular injections, PCA, and epidural analgesics are usually discontinued after 24 to 48 hours. Oral painkillers are then given as necessary.

Will I feel nauseous after surgery?

Effects of anesthesia, the postoperative narcotics, or the surgery itself can cause postoperative nausea. Nausea associated with the anesthetic disappears within the first 6 to 12 hours after surgery. Some of the newer agents used in general anesthesia are less likely to induce nausea. Your anesthesiologist or gynecologist can order anti-nausea medication in the recovery room for you, if necessary. Nausea associated with narcotics can be managed by reducing the dose or changing to a different drug.

Pelvic surgery may cause a temporary decrease in bowel activity. Your bowels are less likely to be affected by laparoscopy and vaginal surgery. After major abdominal surgery, attempting to eat before the bowel is ready will induce nausea and vomiting. Your doctor will wait for signs of bowel activity, evidenced by the passing of gas and sounds audible through a stethoscope, before letting you eat or drink. (This may be the only time in your life that people will be thrilled to hear you pass gas!) Usually fluids are given for 24 hours before solids are attempted. Doctors routinely prescribe anti-nausea medication after major surgery, but you may have to request it. Don't wait until you're retching. If you feel nauseous, ask the nurse for medication.

When can I return to work?

The answer depends on the operation you've had. After minor procedures such as a D&C or hysteroscopy, you can return to work within a day or two. No incisions need to heal, and you really can't create any problems by resuming your work routine. You may experience cramping and bleeding that put you out of commission for a few days, but you'll quickly get back to normal. After laparoscopic surgery, activities can be resumed after several weeks, and you can usually go back to work in two weeks, though it is difficult to give a general answer covering all such cases, since so many operations are now performed laparoscopically.

SURGERY

Following a tubal ligation, your doctor may allow you to return to work within several days. However, you could be out of work for several weeks after a laparoscopic hysterectomy. Most gynecologists will tell you not to work or to do any heavy lifting and pushing for four to six weeks after major vaginal and abdominal surgery so that incisions will have sufficient time to heal. Any activity that increases pressure in the abdomen during the initial healing may increase your risk of developing a hernia. Major reconstructive vaginal surgery also requires restricted activity to ensure adequate healing and to reduce the risk of recurrence.

The nature of your work also influences the decision. If your job is mainly sedentary, you can go back fairly early. On the other hand, jobs that require heavy lifting or other strenuous tasks mandate a longer leave of absence.

Your employer's disability policy may also factor into the equation. Ask your employer (or the director of personnel) about the disability or sick-leave policy. If your time from work is not compensated, you will probably want to return as soon as it is medically safe to do so. However, if the policy is liberal, you may want to extend your absence until you feel stronger.

Your doctor cannot extend your absence unless there is a legitimate medical indication, such as a postoperative complication.

What restrictions will I have after surgery?

Every gynecologist has a philosophy concerning necessary restrictions. You should stay home the first week after major surgery. Take short walks inside or outside the house, and rest, but do not confine yourself to bed. Complete immobility increases your risk of getting blood clots in your veins. It also turns your muscles into mush. You should limit climbing stairs to once or twice daily if possible, and take the steps one at a time while holding on to a handrail. Light cooking that doesn't involve heavy pots and pans is reasonable. Cleaning is out! This is your golden opportunity to get your family involved in those mundane chores that you always did and they took for granted before the surgery. With a little luck (and some good acting), you may even get them to continue helping after you've recovered.

During the second week, it is best if someone else drives you when

you leave the house, and your trips should not be too strenu/
a movie or restaurant. You deserve it. Gradually increase the
walking during the second week but continue to limit heav
pushing. Make your trips to the grocery store brief and let some
else carry the bags.

You can gradually resume normal activities over the next several weeks
and can start driving the car during the third week. You should refrain
from exercise other than walking until six weeks after surgery. After that,
gradually reintroduce exercise and sports. If a particular activity causes
pain, stop. Wait a couple weeks and try again. Activities that involve heavier lifting can slowly be resumed. However, heavy exertions, such as moving furniture or heavy boxes, should be postponed for another few weeks.

Now for the big question: "When can I have sex?" Sexual intercourse can be attempted six weeks following major surgery. After hysterectomy or reconstructive vaginal surgery, wait until your doctor
gives the OK at the postoperative visit, usually six weeks after surgery.
He or she will examine the vagina at that time to see if it has healed
sufficiently. If you have pain during intercourse, stop and wait several weeks. Persistent pain or bleeding during intercourse should be
brought to the attention of your doctor.

There are usually no major restrictions concerning sex after minor
vaginal surgery, such as a D&C or hysteroscopy. However, your doctor
may limit intercourse and use of tampons for one to two weeks.

Restrictions after laparoscopy vary according to the nature of the
operation performed. Simpler procedures, such as laparoscopic tubal
ligation, entail few restrictions. Complicated operations, such as laparoscopically assisted hysterectomies, may carry restrictions similar to
those mentioned for major surgery, although you can often resume normal activity in two to three weeks rather than four to six. Advanced laparoscopic surgery is a relatively new phenomenon, so there is no
consensus yet on how quickly normal activities can be resumed.

What's the difference between a complete hysterectomy and a partial hysterectomy?

A complete hysterectomy removes the entire uterus. It has nothing to
do with the ovaries! We can't emphasize this enough. Often women

think that a complete hysterectomy includes removal of the ovaries. Removal of the ovaries is called oophorectomy.

A partial hysterectomy (also called supracervical hysterectomy) involves the removal of part of the uterus and was a common practice several decades ago. Usually the upper portion of the uterus was removed, including the endometrium and myometrium, but the cervix was left in place. Because the most difficult part of a hysterectomy is the removal of the cervix, if the problem was not related to cancer, doctors usually left the cervix in place. This practice fell out of favor, however, when a significant number of women subsequently developed cervical cancer. Removal of the entire uterus became standard with all hysterectomies.

Recently, in some gynecologic circles, partial hysterectomy is making a comeback. Proponents think that the cervix is important to the normal support of the vagina and bladder. They also postulate that the removal of the cervix may have an adverse impact on sexual and bladder function. Studies in the literature do not resolve this question. Some doctors believe that these hysterectomies are easier and safer, especially when performed laparoscopically. In one such operation, the center of the cervix is "hollowed out" to prevent subsequent cervical cancer. Although this appears to be a reasonable procedure when performed by experienced surgeons, postoperative bleeding affects 10 to 15 percent of women who undergo it.

We don't know if there is an absolute solution to this dilemma. Most gynecologists still think it is best to remove the cervix and recommend complete hysterectomy to prevent future cervical problems, including cervical cancer. If her cervix is left intact, a woman must remember that regular gynecologic visits are absolutely necessary in order to detect any abnormal cervical growth while it is still precancerous and curable.

When I have a hysterectomy, should my ovaries also be removed?

If your ovaries appear normal at surgery, they do not have to be removed during a hysterectomy. However, if you are close to menopause, removal of the ovaries is often recommended. Even after the childbearing years are over, ovaries play an important role. Estrogen made by the ovaries protects bones against osteoporosis and the heart against

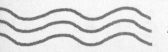

coronary artery disease. Their premature removal places a woman at risk for early onset of these medical problems. Removal of the ovaries will also cause menopausal symptoms such as hot flashes, night sweats, and vaginal dryness.

So why in the world would you want to have your ovaries removed? The answer is plain and simple: avoiding ovarian cancer. You have a 1 in 80 chance of developing this cancer during your lifetime, and although it is not as common as some, it is not rare. Ovarian cancer is difficult to detect early. Only 25 percent of ovarian cancers will still be confined to the ovary when diagnosed. In addition to ovarian cancer, you may also develop benign (noncancerous) ovarian tumors. Even though you are unlikely to die from such a tumor, you will still need additional surgery for its removal.

If you are still far from menopause — less than 40 years old — it is probably best to retain your ovaries, or at least one of them. They will continue to produce hormones for at least ten years. If you are close to menopause (more than 45 years old), it is probably best to remove the ovaries. After all, your hormones can be replaced, which will prevent premature menopause. There's no guarantee that you will feel exactly the same as you did before hormone replacement, but most women are satisfied.

If you have had ovarian problems in the past, such as benign ovarian tumors, or are at increased risk for getting ovarian cancer (see chapter 10), you should certainly consider having your ovaries removed.

How will the doctor perform my hysterectomy?

We're assuming that the decision to perform a hysterectomy has been finalized. If the hysterectomy is performed because of uterine prolapse (see chapter 15), the uterus will be removed vaginally. If it is being extracted to fight cancer, it will probably be removed through an abdominal incision, allowing your doctor to thoroughly explore the pelvis and abdomen to detect any spread of the cancer. An abdominal hysterectomy also permits the removal of lymph nodes if this is deemed necessary. A few doctors are attempting to perform this procedure laparoscopically, but most gynecologic oncologists prefer a larger incision.

Doctors vary in their approach to hysterectomy for benign disease such as bleeding, fibroids, or endometriosis. Many doctors prefer to remove a very large uterus abdominally. A small uterus can usually be removed vaginally. The larger the uterus, the more skill and experience are required to perform the hysterectomy vaginally. A prior history of vaginal deliveries (rather than having delivered no children or delivered them by cesarean section) makes the woman a stronger candidate for vaginal approach, since vaginal childbirth relaxes the ligaments supporting the uterus and allows easier access to it.

Recent advances have made vaginal hysterectomies easier to perform. GnRH agonists (see page 110) can often reduce the size of the uterus, thereby allowing it to be removed vaginally. Advanced laparoscopic techniques have also enabled doctors to perform hysterectomies vaginally that would have previously required an abdominal approach. A laparoscopically assisted vaginal hysterectomy is often used if the ovaries are also to be removed.

A few surgeons perform hysterectomies completely through laparoscopy. However, few doctors have the expertise to perform this operation safely. In laparoscopic hysterectomy, the uterus is removed in tiny pieces through small laparoscopic incisions, possibly extending the duration of surgery beyond reasonable limits.

Will a hysterectomy put me into menopause?

We repeat: Removal of the uterus does not change the production of female hormones. Hormones are produced by the ovaries. If the ovaries are not removed, you will not experience the symptoms related to reduced hormone levels. You will no longer menstruate, but the hormones are still being produced.

A hysterectomy can make it more difficult to detect the onset of menopause. If you have symptoms of menopause, such as hot flashes, night sweats, and vaginal dryness, it may be obvious that the change is occurring. However, 25 percent of women don't experience significant menopausal symptoms. Doctors generally check hormone levels annually for women over age 50 who have undergone hysterectomy to assess ovarian function.

Why do I have to be examined if I have had a hysterectomy?

If your ovaries were not removed during your hysterectomy, it is especially important that you continue with pelvic exams. Ovarian tumors are difficult to detect (see page 142) and usually do not show early symptoms. Pelvic exams are one way to keep a check on the ovaries.

If the ovaries were removed, chances of developing gynecologic problems are certainly decreased, but not eliminated. Although it is uncommon, women can still get vaginal and vulvar cancer. Periodic inspection of these areas is important. The American College of Obstetrics and Gynecology recommends vaginal Pap smears every three to five years following hysterectomy and more frequently if the uterus was removed because of cancer. The doctor will also perform breast and rectal exams during the annual visit. He or she will order necessary screening tests, including mammography. Important topics such as hormone replacement therapy can be discussed at these visits.

If I have an ovarian tumor, does the whole ovary need to be removed?

The short answer is "not always." If you have a benign (noncancerous) cyst or tumor of the ovary, your doctor may be able to perform an ovarian cystectomy. In this procedure, the cyst is removed from the ovary, preserving the remaining normal ovarian tissue. If you have not yet had children or wish to have more, this approach is recommended. If your family is complete, preserving the ovary is not critical, assuming that your other ovary is normal. You need only one ovary to produce your female hormones. Removing the abnormal ovary will not cause premature menopause.

Sometimes technical factors encountered at surgery will dictate whether the entire ovary is removed. If the growth or cyst is exceedingly large, there may not be much normal ovarian tissue to preserve. In that situation, your doctor may elect to remove the whole ovary. The ovary's appearance may reflect the possible presence of cancer. If so, it is safer to remove the entire ovary. Finally, a complication, such as bleeding from the ovary, may require its removal.

SURGERY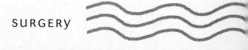

If you are close to menopause (older than age 45), your doctor may also recommend removal of the other ovary even if it appears normal.

Will I need to take hormones after the surgery?

If both of your ovaries are removed, you will abruptly enter menopause, assuming you are premenopausal at the time of surgery. If your hormones are not replaced, you are likely to experience severe hot flashes and night sweats as well as other menopausal symptoms. Most doctors will provide you with hormone replacement therapy to ease this transition. Whether you ultimately continue with hormone replacement depends on many factors (see chapter 13). If one ovary is preserved, hormone replacement is not necessary. If you are menopausal at the time of surgery, no changes will occur after ovarian removal because the ovaries were not functioning before surgery.

Why do I need a catheter for so long after bladder surgery?

Surgery involving the bladder creates inflammation and swelling that can prevent it from emptying itself. A catheter is necessary to drain the urine until the swelling subsides. This period may be as short as one or two days or as long as two to three weeks in duration. The bladder may also be positioned differently after the surgery, which may inhibit it from emptying. With time, it will adjust to its new position.

Doctors vary in their approach to catheterization. Some will place a catheter through the urethra, whereas others will place it in the bladder through the abdominal wall. Doctors may also use intermittent catheterization, a procedure that teaches you how to catheterize yourself. You're probably thinking, "You've got to be kidding!" However, it is surprisingly easy for most women to learn this technique. You can catheterize yourself at periodic intervals (usually every four hours) until you are able to empty your bladder normally.

Why am I losing urine after my bladder surgery?

Perhaps your surgery repaired a "dropped bladder." Or perhaps it corrected stress incontinence. Your catheter is finally removed and you are ready to rejoice. But what's this? All of a sudden you feel as though you

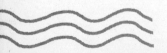

have to run to the bathroom, and the urine starts leaking before you get there. This event was certainly not in the game plan.

Don't be alarmed. This situation is probably only temporary. Bladder surgery and catheterization can temporarily cause bladder instability. Your urgency and frequency of urination and urine loss are probably related to involuntary bladder contractions. As the inflammation from the surgery and catheter subsides, so will your symptoms. In the meantime, they can usually be controlled with medications that will relax the bladder musculature. Your problem may last for only several days, although it is more likely to persist for several weeks. After that time it will usually clear up.

Why do I have pain in my shoulder after laparoscopic surgery?

"OK, what did you guys do? Did you wrench my shoulder?" Have no fear. Your shoulder will be fine. Your mind is playing a trick on you. Gas is used to inflate your abdomen during laparoscopy to provide the visibility necessary for your surgery. At the end of surgery, most of the gas is evacuated, but some always remains in the abdomen, where it rises and irritates the underside of your diaphragm. Your brain interprets this pain as originating in your shoulder. The body absorbs gas fairly quickly, and the shoulder pain will disappear on its own in a day or two.

Why do I have so many incisions on my abdomen?

Don't be deceived into thinking that laparoscopic surgery involves only one incision for the telescopic instrument. Some procedures, such as a tubal ligation or diagnostic laparoscopy, may require only one incision. However, most laparoscopic surgery will involve two to four incisions. As the complexity of the surgery increases, so do the number of incisions. One is used for the laparoscope; the others accommodate surgical instruments. Often, more than one instrument is required simultaneously, so you may have multiple incisions, each one less than one-half inch in size.

Is laparoscopic surgery safer than regular surgery?

This issue is controversial. Doctors who specialize in laparoscopic surgery will often say it's safer than traditional surgery performed through a larger incision. They think the enhanced visibility provided by the laparoscope improves their ability to perform surgery safely. However, most gynecologists are not as facile with laparoscopic surgery as these specialists are. When advanced laparoscopic surgery is attempted by doctors with less experience, the rate of complications may exceed that of the same surgery performed through a traditional approach. Laparoscopic instruments are usually more tedious and cumbersome to use than standard surgical instruments, and in addition, the doctor loses the ability to feel the tissues with his or her hands.

If your doctor has extensive experience in performing a specific laparoscopic operation, he or she can probably perform it safely. Beware of very new laparoscopic procedures. They may sound good, but until all the kinks are worked out, you're probably better off going with a more traditional approach. Although recovery is shorter with laparoscopic surgery, it should not be performed if it might compromise success or increase the possibility of complications.

Can I have laparoscopic surgery as an outpatient?

Most laparoscopic surgery is done in that way. You arrive at the hospital or outpatient surgical facility one to two hours before surgery. After surgery, you spend two to four hours recovering before discharge. If you have excessive pain or nausea and vomiting, your doctor may keep you overnight for observation. Some laparoscopic procedures require a longer postoperative recovery period. An operation such as a laparoscopically assisted vaginal hysterectomy may necessitate a stay of as long as two days. There is tremendous regional variation in the length of stay after laparoscopic surgery. A woman may be discharged as quickly as 8 to 12 hours after this procedure in one region, yet stay two days in another area of the country.

Some doctors perform minor laparoscopic procedures at the office, which provides a more comfortable environment for patients. This setting, however, is usually not equipped to handle major surgical compli-

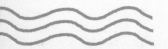

cations. If safety is of paramount importance, you should have your procedure performed at a facility that can expeditiously manage any complication of laparoscopy.

How much pain will I have after laparoscopic surgery?

There is no precise way to gauge how much pain you'll have after surgery. There is usually very little pain after minor laparoscopic procedures such as tubal ligation. Greater pain will follow advanced laparoscopic surgery that uses multiple incisions. Your pain will be less than the discomfort associated with the same procedure performed through a larger, open incision.

Everybody experiences pain differently. However, most of the time you can get adequate relief with oral painkillers. Your doctor should send you home with a prescription for narcotic pain pills. You may be able to get by without them, but keep them on hand just in case.

Can hysteroscopy be done in the office?

Generally, office use of this procedure is confined to diagnostic hysteroscopy. Removal of large polyps and fibroids through the hysteroscope can cause complications that should be managed in a hospital setting.

How much pain and bleeding will I have after hysteroscopy?

Hysteroscopy is usually well tolerated. You can expect to have cramping after the procedure, which can be managed with Tylenol or other non-narcotic analgesics. If the procedure is particularly long in duration or if it involves removing a large polyp or fibroid, your pain may be greater and narcotic analgesics may be necessary. Minor bleeding is typical following hysteroscopy. Removal of large fibroids may cause more bleeding. Pain and bleeding after hysteroscopy should stop over a few days. If you notice progressive worsening of the pain or bleeding, call your doctor; it may be a sign of a complication.

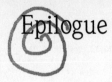

Epilogue

We hope we haven't confused you. Our goal was to provide answers to many of the questions women ask, without getting too technical. You can use this information as a starting point for meaningful discussions with your doctor. He or she can expand on what you have learned and help determine which sections of the book apply to your particular situation.

If you have a problem that is not resolved, it definitely pays to seek another opinion, especially if a specialist deals with the area in question. Keep in mind that not all problems have perfect solutions. Fortunately, medicine is constantly exploring new frontiers and developing new technology. Keep the faith! An answer may be on the horizon.

Finally, make your own health care a priority. We see women who continually nurture family and friends, while ignoring their own emotional and physical needs. Attending to those who mean a lot to you is admirable, but don't forget yourself.

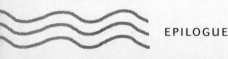

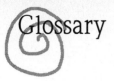

Glossary

The terms listed here are defined in greater detail throughout the book. To find a fuller explanation, consult the index. Italicized words are defined elsewhere in the glossary.

Abscess — a collection of white blood cells (pus).

Adenomyosis — a condition in which the *endometrium* grows into the *myometrium*.

Adhesions — scar tissue that forms after surgery or results from an inflammatory condition.

Afterbirth — see *placenta*.

AIDS (acquired immunodeficiency syndrome) — a disease caused by the HIV virus that destroys *cells* of the immune system (the body's natural defense against disease).

Amenorrhea — total absence of menstruation.

Analgesics — pain relievers.

Anovulation — lack of *ovulation*.

Antibody — a protein produced by the immune system to fight anything foreign that invades the body.

Anus — the opening of the *rectum*.

Areola — the pigmented area surrounding the nipple.

Artificial insemination — the placement of sperm (husband's or donor's) at the opening of the uterus to enhance conception.

Ascites — excessive free fluid in the abdominal cavity.

Aspiration — (1) the withdrawal of fluid from a breast cyst or (2) the accidental inhalation of stomach contents during surgery, bringing them into the lungs.

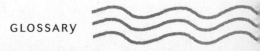

Asymptomatic — not causing symptoms.

Atrophic vaginitis — thinning and inflammation of the vagina, resulting from a lack of *estrogen*.

Bacterial vaginosis — a condition associated with overgrowth of certain bacteria in the *vagina*, corresponding with a decrease in the number of normal vaginal bacteria.

Basal body temperature (BBT) — the body's temperature upon awakening; used in natural family planning and infertility evaluation.

Benign — not cancerous.

B-HCG (beta-human chorionic gonadotropin) — the hormone measured in pregnancy tests, which is produced by the *placenta*.

Biopsy — sampling a piece of *tissue* for diagnosis.

Birth control pills — *oral contraceptive* pills containing *estrogen* and/or *progesterone*.

Bladder — the pelvic organ that serves as the receptacle for urine prior to voiding.

Breast augmentation — a surgical procedure that enlarges the breast.

Breast implants — fluid-filled structures placed under breast tissue or chest wall muscles to augment or reconstruct the breast.

Breast reduction — a surgical procedure that reduces the size of the breast.

Bromocriptine — a substance that inhibits the secretion of prolactin, the *pituitary* hormone normally secreted to induce *lactation* (trade name Parlodel)

CA-125 — a tumor marker for ovarian cancer that can be measured with a blood test.

Candida — a species of yeast that commonly causes vaginal infections.

Capsular contracture — the formation of hard scar tissue around a breast implant.

Catheter — a flexible tube used for drainage.

Cell — the microscopic building block of living matter from which all living plants and animals derive.

Cervical polyp — a benign growth derived from glandular cervical tissue.

Cervicitis — inflammation of the *cervix*.

Cervix — the lower portion of the *uterus* that opens into the *vagina*.

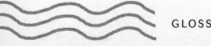

GLOSSARY

Cesarean section — delivery of a baby through an incision made in the wall of the *uterus*.

Chemotherapy — substances that are toxic to living cells and used to treat cancer.

Chlamydia — a sexually transmitted organism that causes uterine and tubal infection.

Chromosome — one of 48 structures in the nucleus of a cell that bears the genetic blueprint.

Clitoris — a sensitive protuberance located just above the vaginal and urethral openings that is important in sexual arousal.

Clomiphene citrate — a substance similar in structure to *estrogen* that is used to stimulate *ovulation* (trade names Clomid and Serophene).

Colposcope — an instrument that magnifies the *cervix* and *vagina* to enhance study of these structures.

Conception — successful attainment of pregnancy.

Condom — a sheath placed over the penis (male condom) or into the vagina (female condom) prior to intercourse for the prevention of pregnancy and *sexually transmitted diseases*.

Condylomata — *genital warts* caused by *human papillomavirus*.

Condylox — a chemical preparation of *podophyllin* used to treat *genital warts*.

Contact dermatitis — a rash that results when a substance contacts the skin and induces an allergic reaction.

Contraception — any process or device that inhibits *conception*.

Cornua — the portion of the *uterus* attached to each *fallopian tube*.

Coronary artery disease — the formation of plaque within the arteries of the heart.

Corpus luteum — the *follicular* structure remaining after *ovulation*, which plays an important role in the secretion of *progesterone*.

Cryotherapy — any treatment that uses a freezing technique.

CT scan (CAT scan) — computerized tomography scan; a type of radiologic scan used to detect certain disorders.

Cyst — a fluid-filled lump or mass.

Cystitis — inflammation of the *bladder*.

Cystocele ("dropped bladder") — descent of the *bladder* into the *vagina* due to inadequate support.

Cystoscopy — use of a telescopic instrument to look into the *bladder* and the *urethra*.

Danazol — a synthesized drug used in the medical treatment of *endometriosis* (trade name Danocrine).

D&C (dilation and curettage) — dilation of the *cervix* followed by *endometrial* scraping, which is used to obtain tissue for purposes of diagnosis.

D&E (dilation and evacuation) — dilation of the *cervix* and removal of pregnancy tissue.

Deep-vein thrombosis (DVT) — blood clot in the deep veins of the legs.

Depo-Provera — an intramuscular preparation of Provera, a synthetic *progesterone*.

Diaphragm — a dome-shaped, flexible device placed in the *vagina* for contraception.

Diuretic ("water pill") — any medication or substance that enhances the kidneys' ability to excrete urine.

Diverticulum — an outpouching from an organ.

Douche — the squirting of liquid into the *vagina*.

Dysmenorrhea — painful *menses*, particularly cramps during the menstrual flow.

Dysplasia — atypical cellular changes that are potentially precancerous.

Ectopic pregnancy — a pregnancy located outside the intrauterine cavity.

Embryo — the earliest stage of life, extending from conception to approximately the end of the second month of life.

Endometrial — pertaining to the *endometrium*.

Endometrial biopsy — passage of a small catheter into the *uterus* to obtain a sample of the *endometrium*.

Endometrial cancer — cancer of the interior glandular lining of the *uterus*.

Endometrial polyp — a benign growth derived from the *endometrium* that projects into the uterine cavity.

Endometriosis — a condition in which *endometrial* tissue is located outside the *uterus*.

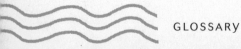

Endometrium — the glandular lining inside the *uterus*. It thickens throughout the menstrual cycle and is shed during the menstrual period.

Enterocele — *herniation* between the walls of the *rectum* and *vagina*.

Estrogen — the fundamental "female" hormone responsible for secondary sexual characteristics. It also plays important roles in maintaining bone density and preventing *coronary artery disease*.

Excisional biopsy — breast biopsy in which the entire area in question is removed.

Fallopian tubes — the two tubes extending from the *uterus* to the *ovaries* (one on each side), which allow for the transport of sperm and eggs between the uterus and ovaries.

Familial — affecting multiple individuals within a family, usually as a result of genetic inheritance.

Fertilization — the impregnation of an egg by a sperm.

Fibrocystic breast disease — the development of cystic glands and fibrotic nodules within breast tissue.

Fibroid — a smooth muscle tumor that develops in the muscular wall of the *uterus*.

Fimbria — fingerlike projections from the end of the *fallopian tube*, which play an important role in picking up the egg from the *ovary* after *ovulation*.

Follicle — a small fluid-filled structure in the *ovary* containing an egg, also responsible for the secretion of the female hormones.

Follicular — pertaining to the *follicle*.

Fundus — the upper portion of the *uterus*, excluding the *cervix*.

Galactorrhea — leakage of milk from the breasts that does not occur during pregnancy or nursing.

Gamete — the primary cell involved in reproduction (egg or sperm).

Gamete intrafallopian transfer (GIFT) — transfer of an egg from the *ovary* to a healthy portion of the *fallopian tube*.

Gene — a piece of genetic material on a *chromosome* that regulates a specific function.

Genitalia — the organs of the reproductive system.

Genital warts — warts located on the external genitals, *vagina*, or *cervix*, caused by *human papillomavirus*; also called *condylomata* and *venereal warts*.

GnRH agonists — a group of substances that inhibit the secretion of *gonadotropins* from the *pituitary gland*.

Gonadotropins — signals sent to the *ovaries* from the *pituitary gland* that regulate ovarian function.

Gonorrhea — a sexually transmitted bacterium that can cause uterine and tubal infection.

"G spot" (the Grafenberg spot) — an area located on the vaginal wall purported to create vaginal orgasm.

Hepatitis B — one of several hepatitis viruses that may be sexually transmitted and cause liver infection, liver failure, or cancer.

Hepatitis B immune globulin — antibodies that combat *hepatitis B*, which can be administered shortly after exposure to hepatitis B in order to prevent infection.

Hepatitis B vaccine — a vaccine against *hepatitis B*.

Herniation — protrusion of an *organ* or part of an organ through weak support tissue.

Herpes simplex — a sexually transmittable virus that causes oral and genital herpes infections.

Human immunodeficiency virus (HIV) — a sexually transmitted virus responsible for causing AIDS.

Human papillomavirus (HPV) — a sexually transmittable virus that causes *genital warts* and can induce cervical *dysplasia*.

Hysterectomy — surgical removal of the *uterus*.

Hysterosalpingogram (HSG) — an x-ray of the *uterus* and *fallopian tubes* taken after the injection of radiographic dye into the *uterus*.

Hysteroscopy — a means of looking into the *uterus* with a telescopic instrument (a hysteroscope) inserted through the *vagina* and *cervix*.

Hymen — a ring of tissue partly covering the opening of the *vagina*.

Incontinence — involuntary loss of urine.

Insemination — the depositing of semen into the *vagina*.

Interferons — naturally occurring proteins that the body uses to fight viruses.

Interstitial cystitis — a chronic, inflammatory *bladder* disorder.

Intraductal papilloma — a noncancerous growth in a breast duct.

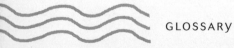

GLOSSARY

Intravenous (within the vein) — a term used to describe anything administered directly into the bloodstream.

Introl — a removable device placed in the *vagina* to prevent *stress incontinence*.

In vitro fertilization (IVF) — a process that includes three steps: (1) removal of eggs from the *ovary*, (2) fertilization of the eggs with sperm in a laboratory, and (3) reintroduction of one or more *embryos* into the *uterus*.

IUD (intrauterine device) — a device placed in the *uterus* to prevent pregnancy.

Kegel exercises — exercises that tighten and strengthen the pelvic muscles.

Labia — the "lips," or folds of tissue, located just outside the opening of the *vagina*.

Lactation — the production of breast milk.

Lactobacillus — the dominant bacterium in the *vagina*, under normal conditions.

Laparoscopically assisted vaginal hysterectomy — a *vaginal hysterectomy* assisted by laparoscopic surgery.

Laparoscopy — a means of looking into the abdomen and pelvis through a telescopic instrument (a laparoscope) inserted through a small abdominal incision. More than one incision may be required for some procedures.

Laparotomy — surgery performed through a large abdominal incision.

Laser — a high-energy beam.

LEEP (loop electrosurgical excision procedure) — a procedure in which a wire loop conducting electrical energy is used to excise cervical tissue.

Libido — sex drive.

Lipoma — a noncancerous fatty tumor.

Lumpectomy — removal of a cancerous lump, while still preserving the remaining breast tissue.

Lymph nodes — oval or round nodules within the lymphatic system, which handles tissue fluids.

Malignant — cancerous.

Mammogram — an x-ray of the breast.

GLOSSARY

Mastitis — inflammation of the breast, usually from bacterial infection.

Melanoma — a skin cancer derived from pigment-producing cells, usually referred to as malignant melanoma.

Menarche — the time of the first menstrual flow or period.

Menopause — permanent cessation of the *menses*.

Menses — the periodic discharge of blood and *endometrial* tissue from the uterus.

Menstrual cycle — the interval between *menses*, consisting of two phases: an early, or follicular, and a late, or luteal, phase.

Menstrual period — same as *menses*.

Metastasis — the spread of cancer beyond the organ of origin.

Minipill — refers to *oral contraceptives* that contain only *progesterone*.

Mittelschmerz — severe pelvic pain experienced in the middle of the *menstrual cycle*, caused by *ovulation*.

Monilia — generic term for a group of fungi that commonly cause vaginal infections.

Mucosa — the inside lining of the *vagina*.

Myolysis — a means of shrinking fibroids by inserting a needle or probe and applying electrical energy or by freezing.

Myomectomy — removal of a *fibroid* from the *uterus*.

Myometrium — the muscular wall of the *uterus*.

Natural family planning — preventing pregnancy without using "artificial" contraception.

Neoplasm — a growth of tissue that can be cancerous or noncancerous.

Norplant — flexible rods impregnated with *progesterone* that are implanted under the skin of the arm and slowly release *progesterone* for contraception.

Oligomenorrhea — infrequent menstruation.

Omentum — a sheet of fatty tissue that overlays the intestines.

Oncologist — a doctor who specializes in treating cancer.

Oophorectomy — removal of the *ovaries*.

Oral contraceptives — pills containing *estrogen* and/or *progesterone*, designed to prevent pregnancy.

Organ — any part of the body performing a specific function.

Orgasm — the climax of sexual response.

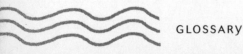

GLOSSARY

Osteoporosis — the loss of calcium from bones; thinning of the bones.

Ovarian cystectomy — surgical removal of a *cyst* from the *ovary*.

Ovaries — the two reproductive glands in the female that contain eggs and produce the female hormones.

Ovulation — the rupture of a *follicle* in the *ovary* at midcycle, which releases an egg.

Paget's disease — a type of skin cancer that may be found on the *vulva*.

Palpable — able to be felt with the hands.

Pancreatic — relating to the pancreas, an organ that produces enzymes necessary for the digestion of food.

Pap smear — a test in which cells from the *cervix* are placed on a slide for analysis; most commonly used in screening for cervical cancer.

Partial hysterectomy — surgical removal of the *uterus*, while still preserving the *cervix*.

Pectoralis muscles — the two large muscles extending across the front of the chest, beneath the breasts.

Pelvic inflammatory disease (PID) — bacterial infection of the pelvic organs, including the *uterus* and *fallopian tubes*.

Pelvic prolapse — general term referring to descent of the pelvic organs (*uterus, bladder, rectum*) due to inadequate support.

Pergonal — a purified preparation of *gonadotropins* used to artificially stimulate the *ovary*.

Perianal — referring to the area around the *anus*.

Perimenopausal — the time preceding *menopause* that is associated with declining function of the *ovaries*.

Perineum — the area between the *vagina* and *anus*.

Pessary — a rubber device placed into the *vagina* to support pelvic organs.

Phytoestrogen — a plant compound with *estrogenic* activity.

Pituitary gland — a gland located at the base of the brain that secretes hormonal signals, regulating ovarian function.

Placenta — the organ that connects the fetus (by its umbilical cord) to the mother. It provides nutrition to the baby from the mother. After delivery, it is expelled as the "afterbirth."

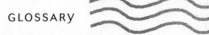

PMS (premenstrual syndrome) — physical and emotional symptoms that occur before the *menstrual period*.

Podophyllin — a caustic chemical used in the treatment of *genital warts*.

Polycystic ovaries — a condition in which the *ovaries* accumulate multiple *follicular cysts*.

Polyp — a growth of *tissue* that projects outward from a surface, such as the lining of the *uterus*, *cervix*, or *vagina*.

Progesterone — the "second female hormone." Made by the *ovary* and *placenta*, it is necessary for supporting pregnancy and plays an important role in balancing the effects of *estrogen* on the *endometrium*.

Prolactin — the hormone responsible for inducing *lactation*.

Prolapse — an organ falling downward.

Prostaglandins — a group of substances that induce contraction of smooth muscle. They are released naturally from the *endometrium*.

Pudendal neuralgia — pain in the pelvic region, caused by disease or injury of the pudendal nerve.

Radical hysterectomy — removal of the *uterus* and its surrounding *tissue* and *lymph nodes*.

Reanastomosis — rejoining two parts of a *fallopian tube* that has been severed.

Rectocele — bulging of the *rectum* into the *vagina* due to inadequate support.

Rectum — the end of the large bowel that serves as a receptacle for stool prior to its evacuation.

RU-486 (mifepristone) — an antiprogestational agent used to induce early termination of pregnancy.

Saline solution (salt water) — the foundation of most intravenous solutions.

Sebaceous glands — the tiny glands in the skin that secrete an oily substance.

SERM (selective estrogen receptor modulator) — a drug that mimics the effects of *estrogen* in some organs, while blocking it in others.

Sexually transmitted disease (STD) — any disease that can be spread through a sexual encounter.

Silicone — a plastic made from silicon.

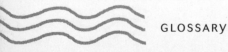

GLOSSARY

Speculum — a device inserted into the *vagina* that opens to allow inspection of the vagina and *cervix*.

Spermicide — a chemical that kills sperm; used in contraceptive creams, gels, and suppositories.

Sterilization — a procedure that permanently renders one incapable of *conception*.

Stress incontinence — see *urinary stress incontinence*.

Thrombophlebitis — inflammation of the veins associated with blood clots.

Tissue — a collection of similar cells.

Trichloroacetic acid (TCA) — a chemical used in the treatment of *genital warts*.

Trichomonas — a single-cell parasite that causes vaginal infections and is sexually transmitted.

Triglycerides — fats that circulate in the bloodstream.

Tubal pregnancy — a pregnancy that has become implanted in the *fallopian tube*.

Tumor — generic term used to denote a growth or *neoplasm*, which can be cancerous or noncancerous.

Ultrasound — high-frequency sound waves used to produce scans.

Ureters — the tubes connecting the kidneys to the *bladder*.

Urethra — a tube that extends from the *bladder* to the body's exterior.

Urethral meatus — the opening of the *urethra*, which is located immediately above the opening of the *vagina*.

Urgency incontinence — loss of urine associated with an urge to empty the *bladder*.

Urinary retention — excessive retention of urine in the *bladder*.

Urinary stress incontinence — sudden loss of urine associated with sudden increases in pressure within the abdomen, which may occur in activities such as running, jumping, laughing, coughing, and sneezing.

Uterine descensus — the descent of the *uterus* into the *vagina* due to inadequate support.

Uterus — the womb; a muscular organ located in the pelvis, in which the fertilized egg develops into a baby. The uterus is composed of a lower part, referred to as the *cervix* (which opens into the vagina), and an upper part, referred to as the *fundus*.

Vagina — the tubular structure extending from the *uterus* to the *vulva*; also referred to as the birth canal during delivery.

Vaginal hysterectomy — surgical removal of the *uterus* through the *vagina*.

Vaginal vault prolapse — a protrusion of the *vagina* due to inadequate support.

Vaginismus — painful spasm of the *vagina* during intercourse.

Vaginitis — inflammation of the *vagina*.

Vas deferens — the tubes that carry sperm from the testicles to the penis.

Venereal warts — *genital warts* induced by a sexually transmitted virus.

Vestibule — the area at the opening of the *vagina*, located between the *labia*.

Vestibulitis — an inflammatory condition limited to the *vestibule*.

VIN (vulvar intraepithelial neoplasia) — abnormal vulvar skin exhibiting potentially precancerous changes.

Vulva — the *tissue* surrounding the opening of the *vagina* that includes the inner and outer "lips" of the vagina.

Vulvectomy — surgical removal of the *vulva*.

Vulvitis — inflammation of the *vulva*.

Vulvodynia — vulvar pain, often of unknown origin.

Yeast — a form of fungus that may cause vaginal and vulvar infections.

Zygote — an egg that has been fertilized by a sperm.

Zygote intrafallopian transfer (ZIFT) — the transfer of a fertilized egg into a healthy portion of a *fallopian tube*.

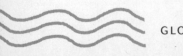

GLOSSARY

Index

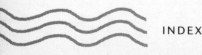

INDEX

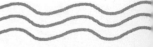

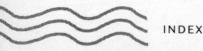

INDEX

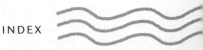

INDEX

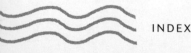

INDEX

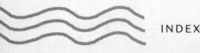

INDEX

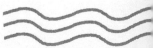

INDEX

INDEX

235

INDEX